AT WAR WITH PARKINSON'S DISEASE

At War With Parkinson's Disease

JAMES JOSEPH PELOSI

AT WAR WITH PARKINSON'S DISEASE

DEDICATION

I dedicate this book to my mother, Mrs. Dorothy Rinderknecht Pelosi (1924 – 2010) and to her sister, Mrs. Katherine Rinderknecht Daspro (1920 – 1997) both of whom battled Parkinson's disease and fought a good fight.

I dedicate this book also to Doctor Engineer Valfredo Zolesi, Ph.D., Founder, Owner and President of Kayser Italia S.r.l., Italy's premier independent, family-owned aerospace system engineering company whom I have known for 15 years. Now in the sixth year, he continues to battle Parkinson's disease. He is an inspiration to his family, his company team members, professional associates and me.

I wrote this book hoping that the contents might give courage and strength to those who are battling this disease and to their families, friends and care providers who are with them and who are supporting them.

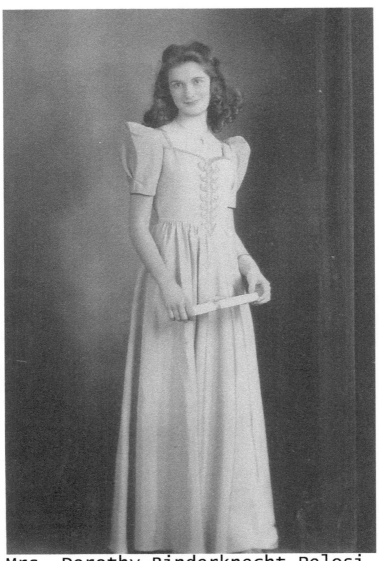

Mrs. Dorothy Rinderknecht Pelosi
High School Graduation, 1943.

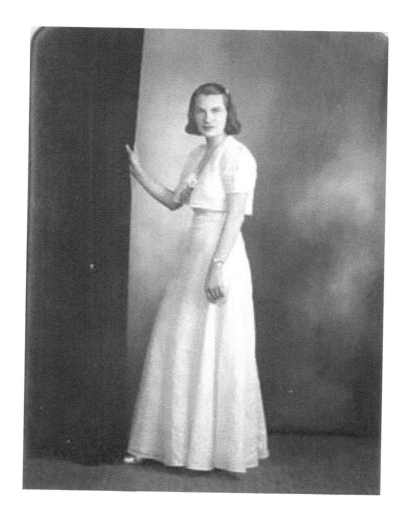

Mrs. Katherine Rinderknecht Daspro
High School Graduation, 1938.

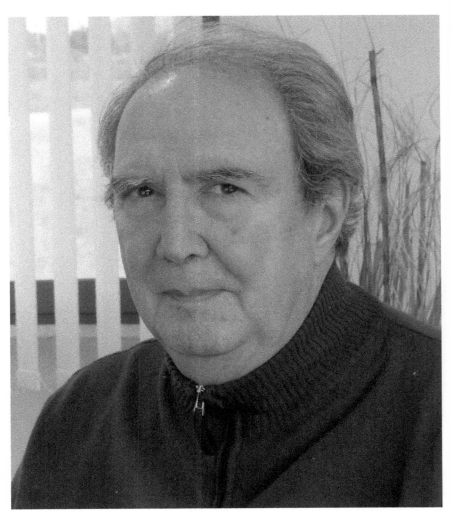

Doctor Engineer Valfredo Zolesi
Founder, President, Kayser Italia Srl

JAMES JOSEPH PELOSI

CONTENTS

APPENDICIES

OTHER BOOKS BY THIS AUTHOR

Normandy to Berlin: The Trek to Honor the Legacies.

The book, *Normandy to Berlin: The Trek to Honor the Legacies,* describes the author's 895-mile solo walk between Omaha Beach, Normandy, France and the Brandenburg Gate, Berlin, Germany in 2014 to honor all veterans. Available at amazon.com.

ACKNOWLEDGMENTS

This was a difficult book for me to write. My first book, *"Normandy to Berlin: The TREK to Honor the Legacies,"* was much easier. Before writing that book, I already knew the history of the four Legacy events: the Start of World War I in 1914; The Allied invasion of Normandy, France in 1944; The End of the Berlin Airlift in 1949; and, The Fall of the Berlin Wall in 1989, from history classes which I took in high school and at the Military Academy, and from living 15 years in Europe, (four of which were in Berlin). I also kept a detailed journal of the 74-day TREK, and recorded daily each evening the highlights of my experiences during the walk between the 59 cities from Normandy, France to Berlin, Germany. I met many people and made many new friends with whom I still have contact.

For this book, I only knew the experience of my mother's sister who suffered from Parkinson's disease and other possible Parkinson's-related debilities, and what I had read from much of the available literature about Parkinson's using sources in the library and on the internet. Once my mother came to live with me in September 2000, I was too busy with work and with her care to keep a daily journal. I did continue to read as much as I could about the disease and my sisters helped me with information. But instead of a journal, I had only records of doctors' visits, medical examinations, Medicare and hospital billings, insurance statements, police reports, court records, ticket stubs from festivals, concerts and plays, and archived letters and memorandums which constituted the sources for much of the material in this book.

Here I wish to express my appreciation to those persons who helped me and the organizations which supported me throughout the 10 years that I cared for my mother as a person living with Parkinson's disease. I am very much thankful for their help.

Ms. Helen Irene Schenck, has been my most valuable supporter for the past 30 years. When I traveled, she helped maintain my home, collect my mail, and provided loving care for my two dogs. She hosted my mother and me in her Melbourne, Florida home when we traveled from Texas to Florida to visit my sisters. She came to Texas to spend holidays with us. She reviewed the entire text of this narrative, and she contributed many of the details about events which I had forgotten. She continues to make the best home-made brownies that I ever have eaten.

My sisters, Kathy Pelosi (deceased) and Janet Diamond, provided the support that could come only from a daughter. Their care, affection and love always uplifted our mother's spirit. She was continuously happy when they were together and while they were spoiling her with attention. When we needed them, they always were there for us.

My two first cousins also helped me with

their contributions. John Daspro related his mother Kate's stories about growing up with my mother and the good times and not-so-good times which they experienced. He also provided some new information about their father, our grandfather who always was fun company for us.

My cousin Louis Pelosi provided me the details about his medical event which compromised a portion of his brain and may triggered an urge to eat ice cream. He is now fully recovered.

After September 2000, I either could have continued to work with NASA or could have been a full-time care provider. I was able to continue my work and provide care only because of the outstanding support I received from the five women who worked as home health care aides with us for 10 years. Each woman was unique in personality and slightly different with the care routine which she provided my mother. But, without exception, all five women were attentive, caring, compassionate, considerate, gentle and, most of all, loving. I am indebted to the support from Ms. Emma Agee, Ms. Mary Davis, Mrs. Lynn Clarkson, Ms. Sharon Gadson, and Mrs. Deborah Schooley.

Our neighbors made our lives more meaningful and happier. The Garan and Arnold families, our next-door neighbors for most of our 10 years together, were as helpful to me and as loving to my mother as if we were family. Whenever we were together, for yard parties, birthday parties, holiday parties, school sporting events or concerts, we did feel as

vi

if we were a part of their family. The five children were especially kind, gracious and respectful. The support that Carmel Garan provided us during times of medical emergencies and throughout the end-of-life week helped me greatly, a demonstration of compassion and love that I always remember when I count my blessings.

I am a graduate of the United States Military Academy at West Point with the "Proud and Free" Class of 1973. Among my classmates in the Clear Lake area where I lived while caring for my mother were Colonel Bill McArthur, a NASA astronaut, and his wife Cindy, a NASA employee in the Education Office. My work at NASA supported them both. They gave me great personal support for my work. Our classmate, Major Jack Whalen, and his wife Vita also lived in Clear Lake. We attended the same church, and Jack and Vita hosted us at their home. My time with both families provided me great encouragement with everything that I was doing.

A graduate of West Point's Class of 1969, is Dr. Charles Whatton, who became my mother's dentist. His wife Jennifer worked as his scheduler and receptionist. We became very good friends. Dr. Whatton and his staff always made our regular visits to his office a pleasant and enjoyable experience, something rare to be said about a visit to the dentist.

In the Medical Professional complex, next door to Dr. Whatton, was Dr. Aguilar, my mother's physician and his nurse, Michele. For eight years, they were the primary care providers for both of us. Both Dr. Aguilar and Michele were compassionate professionals. My mother remained healthy because of the regular care which they provided to us.

I am thankful to the pastors and their staff at St. Clare of Assisi Roman Catholic Church. We were supported by Fathers John, Dominic, Bob and Vincent. Each had a different style ministering to his parishioners. My mother accepted them equally, having no favorite among them. Her funeral Mass was a very respectful and solemn ceremony. The staff provided a reception and full meal for everyone following the Mass, which I did not expect. St. Clare's was among the better parishes of which I have been a member.

For me, the most exciting part of living in Houston and the Clear Lake area was NASA and the astronaut community at the Johnson Space Center. As a former military officer and pilot I had much in common with many of the military astronauts. I enjoyed my work supporting the experiments which they demonstrated on orbit and spending time with them off-duty. My mother and I met many of these highly talented individuals and their families at functions for the crew and at events within Clear Lake. I am grateful for my association with the crew and their families and especially thankful for the attendance of eight astronauts and their families at my mother's funeral.

I am as grateful for my fellow NASA engineers with whom I worked for 12 years in Clear Lake. Many had met my mother. All were exceptional in the attention that they showed to her. I left many good friends behind when I moved away.

I wish to thank the support staff at NASA's Ellington Field for the special parking and seating which they provided us when my mother and I attended the crew return ceremony following a mission in space. Because of my mother's disability status, we were privileged to park and sit in an area reserved for the crew, their families and guests. We both were proud to welcome the crews home from their spaceflight missions.

The Harris County, Texas Sheriff's Department deserves special recognition for its support. On two occasions they responded to incidents during which my mother's life was threatened. They were diligent in their pursuit of the evil-doers, captured them all, and added to the testimony against them when they were tried and then found guilty. Five of five persons tried and convicted went to prison. No such thing as "Catch and Release" in the state of Texas.

My final acknowledgement is to the very professional in-flight staff of United Airlines: the pilots and the cabin crews. My mother and I made seven flights nationally with United and every one of those flights was a pleasure. The pilots and their crews maintain and generate the business for United. I continue to support them and fly with them.

AT WAR WITH PARKINSON'S DISEASE

"Of the events of war, I have not ventured to write from any chance information, nor according to any notion of my own. I have described nothing but what I saw myself, or learned from others of whom I made the most careful and particular inquiry. The task was a laborious one because witnesses of the same circumstance gave different accounts. My narrative may be disappointing. But if he who desires to have before his eyes a true picture. . .shall pronounce what I have written to be useful, then I shall be satisfied.

Thucydides.

"Peloponnesian War, Volume 1" 400 B.C.

FOREWARD

I titled this book *At War with Parkinson's Disease* because, from the early onset of symptoms to the shock of a confirmed diagnosis through the days, weeks, months and years of struggle to manage and control Parkinson's disease, the experience is a battle. Like a soldier in combat, the Parkinson's patient must know himself and know his enemy. He must have as much information as possible about what threatens his life. He must be surrounded and assisted by persons who have the same or more information about this enemy and who fully support him emotionally, physically, medically, logistically and professionally without hesitation, anytime and anywhere.

Chapter 4, "Signs and Symptoms," begins with the statement: "Many people know from reading history and from viewing documentaries about war that the service member in combat who is fighting a battle or who is closest to the battlefield is the most accurate and reliable source for information about what is happening or what has happened." Continuing, I write that: "I have the same sense of awareness for the signs and symptoms of Parkinson's disease. The individual himself or his spouse, companion with whom he may be living, children, other close family members, and neighbors and coworkers who are in frequent contact with someone usually are the first to detect the signs and symptoms."

What follows is a narrative which describes what I learned about Parkinson's disease during the 10 years between 2000 and 2010 when I cared in my home for my mother as a person with Parkinson's, and the eight years since her death as I researched material for this book. It is my opinion that an intelligent man who has had no experience with something is really of less value than the man who has "been there, done that." I could have paraphrased what I have quoted above from Thucydides but, with respect to my mother and me, I could not have made a better statement about my work, our experiences and our battle. I hope that the reader will find the information useful.

AT WAR WITH PARKINSON'S DISEASE

"Love begins by taking care of the closest ones - the ones at home."

Mother Teresa.

1. INTRODUCTION

Life Has Its Duties.

In September 2014, I wrote and published a 316-page book entitled, *Normandy to Berlin: The Trek to Honor the Legacies.* I began the first chapter of that book with a four-word sentence, "All life is precious." I wrote the book as a tribute to the American and Allied veterans of the military who served and who fought in both World Wars, who supported the Berlin Airlift and who helped bring about the fall of the Berlin Wall and the reunification of Germany. Millions died during the two World Wars. Thousands died during the Cold War.

Most of what we know about ourselves and our abilities to meet, understand, overcome or accept the challenges which confront us daily we learn as we proceed through life. We seek happiness for ourselves, and we do that with the love and the help provided by our families, our closest friends, very often our neighbors and occasionally our coworkers. We learn at a very early age that much of anyone's personal happiness often is related to his emotional, spiritual and physical well-being.

We feel empathy for those among us who were born deformed, diseased, disabled, blind, deaf or otherwise handicapped. Similarly, we sympathize and feel compassion for the plight of the elderly and their struggles to care and provide for themselves as they age, as their strength and senses diminish, as their mobility becomes restricted and as they experience age-related illnesses and suffer injuries such as a broken hip.

But we have evolved to die. Knowing that, and more than only wishing for a peaceful death, most of us wish not to suffer as we age. Most of us also do not want to become a burden for anyone who may have to care for us when we are unable to care for ourselves. Families who are forced to make decisions about their loved ones' debilitating status struggle to find solutions which are loving, caring, practical, affordable and, perhaps most importantly, conscionable.

Issues such as these form the basis for the purpose of this book in which I describe my sentiments and experiences during the 10 years that I enjoyed serving as the primary care provider for my mother, Dorothy Rinderknecht Pelosi, 27 years my senior, who lived with

Parkinson's disease. Over those years, I did for her as an adult what she did for me as an infant and toddler: feeding, tending to hygiene, bathing, dressing, entertaining, protecting and loving. Caring for her taught me the most I've ever learned from anyone about love, life and living.

I am a Baby Boomer, born in 1951, at the earlier part of a Generation which dates its births between about 1946 after the end of World War II and the early 1960's before the start of the US involvement in Vietnam. Our parents were part of what American television journalist Tom Brokaw and others have described as "The Greatest Generation," those men and women who fought and who worked to help win World War II.

The street on which I first lived when my parents settled in Nassau County on Long Island, New York was a cul-de-sac of homes with 12 on either side of the street and four in a semi-circle at the dead end. After my family arrived, there were 26 families with 48 school-age children enrolled in the local parochial or public grade schools, high school or college.

All the children were healthy, active, played sports and games, and stayed outdoors all day during the summer until we were summoned inside by our mothers for dinner or by one of our parents after it was dark and the hour was late. The boys found jobs whenever and wherever anyone would hire them: delivering newspapers, working as local store clerks, washing cars, raking leaves, shoveling snow, even as Altar Boys at St. Thomas the Apostle Roman Catholic Church. (Serving at one marriage, one baptism or one funeral Mass netted an Altar Boy $5.00, which was more money earned from working in two hours indoors than any boy earned in one week outdoors in all kinds of weather delivering newspapers.)

Only two mothers worked. They were those unfortunate young women who had lost their husbands, the primary bread winners, unexpectedly early. The rest of the mothers stayed busy as stay-at-home moms very familiar with almost everything that their children and their neighbors' children were doing when they were out and about in the neighborhood. All the mothers knew all the children by their first names. All but one of the mothers was very well known to us children.

Stephen's Mother.

There was one mother who none of us children knew very well. Some of us children did not know her at all. She was the mother of Stephen, one of my neighbors and friends at school. We lived six homes apart on the same street.

Stephen was born eight days before me in 1951. He had a brother perhaps four years his junior and a sister younger by perhaps six years.

Stephen and I were closest as friends during our high school years between 1965 and 1969. Together we suffered through many of the same classes, supported many of the same student organizations, attended most of the school and class functions, and competed for the friendship and attention of many of the same girls.

We were about 300 miles apart on the east coast during our college years between 1969 and 1973. Afterwards we kept in contact for perhaps another 20 years.

Like my father, Stephen's father also was a World War II veteran. He served in the Army as a ground soldier entering Europe at or shortly after the Allied invasion at Normandy, France in June 1944 as a Private, and leaving Europe a year and a half later at the end of the war having earned promotions up every rank to the most senior enlisted grade.

After Stephen told me that I said, "Your father must have been quite a skilled, professional and courageous soldier."

He answered, "I think that the casualty rates had a lot more to do with it."

Regardless, Stephen's father was a very smart man. After the war, I think that he went back to school on the GI bill. He received an education and additional training as an accountant. He was working in that capacity at a county position when his wife became sick. As a result of her illness he became the primary care provider for her and their three children. While doing so, he worked from home.

Stephen's mother, a certified Registered

Nurse, had received a diagnosis of early onset Parkinson's disease shortly after the birth of his sister, the family's third child.

Stephen, his brother and sister, and I and my two younger sisters all were very close in age. Still very young children, none of the three of us in my family knew what was wrong with Stephen's mother. I do not believe that I ever understood anything my parents said and tried to explain when they described her condition and status to me.

Very early after her diagnosis and often when I came calling for Stephen at his home his mother would greet me at the front door. She would address me by name, invite me inside her home to the living room, and tell me, "Please wait here James while I find Stephen," when she left me to find and summon her son.

Her voice was very quiet. I think that when she spoke she sounded as if she had a slight stutter. When she walked away from me to find her son, I noticed that she had a slow, seemingly slightly imbalanced shuffle. I also noticed that on the end table next to the sofa on which she had been sitting and reading were what may have been small bottles of medication.

Because I could not understand her very well I did not initiate any conversation. When she did speak to me it was very hard for me emotionally to tell her sometimes that I did not understand her. She was close in age to my mother. After visits like this, I always wondered how difficult life must have been for this family, especially for my friend Stephen.

Stephen's father, lovingly demonstrating a faithfulness to his marriage vows, was a hero. He kept his family together in their home from which he worked. He stayed with and beside his wife with complete fidelity to their marriage vows. On the first floor of their two-story home he converted a room next to the master bedroom into his home office. The master bedroom had only one matrimonial bed. Also, on the first floor he converted a second room into a spa with an oversized whirlpool bath. He shopped for the groceries, made the meals, cared for the children, ensured that they studied to receive their religious education and the Sacraments, did the yardwork, answered the door at Halloween for the Trick or Treaters, decorated the home at Christmas, piled presents under the Christmas tree.

Yet somehow, he still found time to ride his bicycle in the early evenings and to play golf on the occasional weekend and holidays with my father. He was ever upbeat, always smiling, quick-witted, and gregarious. Stephen, as I remember him, is much in his image.

Occasionally they had nursing and physical therapy care at home. But I never knew anything about the services or the frequency.

As the Parkinson's seized greater hold of her mind and body, Stephen's mother became less mobile and more comfortable with her care and daily routine in their bedroom. I and my family very rarely saw her. Then, surprisingly, one glorious late spring or early summer day on the weekend, my father came home to tell us that he had seen Stephen's parents sitting together outside the front of their home enjoying the sunshine and fresh air. My parents left our home to walk down the street and sit with them.

At dinner that evening, my father told us that Stephen's mother had received some new medication which targeted the Parkinson's and its symptoms. Early results indicated that the medication was proving effective. There seemed to be a marked improvement in her condition. At school the next week, Stephen told me much the same information. He gave the name "Levodopa" to this new medicine. We all hoped and prayed for a miracle.

But it was not granted.

I was away from the neighborhood on duty with the Army when my parents informed me that Stephen's mother had died. I know that I wrote a long letter to his father. I cannot remember how I expressed myself to Stephen. Upon reflection, I wish that I had known then even half what I learned and know now maybe 40 years later. I could have been a better neighbor and a better friend.

"Living with an incurable disease like Parkinson's is very different from living with a terminal illness. This is a disease you're going to live with for a long time."

Connie Carpenter-Phinney, Olympic Gold Medalist.

2. WHAT IS THIS DISEASE

Overview.

Parkinson's disease is an age-related, degenerative brain disease. It is the second most common disorder of this type after Alzheimer's disease. A person who has been diagnosed with Parkinson's disease has a brain which gradually loses more than 50 percent and as much as 80 percent of the cells which produce the chemical dopamine.

Dopamine is a neurotransmitter which stimulates motor neurons in the central nervous system. It serves as the agent which helps to transmit nerve impulses that control movement and coordination and facilitate other physical and mental functions within our body.

Approximately one in 350 persons within the American population has a diagnosis for Parkinson's disease. That represents between one and two percent of the general population, and between two and four percent of the population over the age of 60. The average age for someone of either sex who becomes symptomatic and who receives this diagnosis is around age 60.

In general, there are three age-related categories for the onset for persons with Parkinson's disease. The first, Juvenile Parkinson's, is extremely rare and has its onset in early childhood. Next, is Early-Onset Parkinson's which may manifest symptoms as early as the 20's but more frequently in the 30's and 40's. Finally, the third category, with which we are most familiar, is Late-Onset Parkinson's which becomes symptomatic usually at or after age 60.

The symptoms for Parkinson's disease develop slowly over months and progressively worsen over months and years. They have a variety of characteristics such as tremors, difficulty starting movements, slowness and shuffling while walking, impaired balance, rigidity of the limbs and general stiffness.

Over time, Parkinson's will affect all the muscles of a person's body. Several years usually pass from the onset of symptoms until conditions of serious disability and several more years until death. The symptoms, their onset, the order in which they appear, their intensity and duration vary greatly between persons with the disease. Chapter 4 describes the signs and symptoms of Parkinson's disease in more detail.

The majority of persons with Parkinson's disease manage their symptoms with medication, daily routine of diet, exercise and physical therapy, and regular evaluations with their doctors. Medication serves only to ameliorate the symptoms. There is no medication which can halt the progression of this disease.

Surprisingly, Parkinson's disease is not a killer disease. The life expectancy for people with Parkinson's disease usually is about the same for people without the disease.

Longevity becomes an issue only in the advanced stages of Parkinson's disease when problems from symptoms further compromise someone. For example, poor balance and difficulty walking may result in falls, broken bones, and hospitalization which weaken the body, and rehabilitation and physical therapy which can be stressful. Problems with eating, chewing, and swallowing may result in aspirating food particles that compromise the lungs and may cause pneumonia which is an especially serious condition for any senior whose system already is compromised severely.

There is an expression within the medical and nursing communities which is, "You do not die from Parkinson's disease. You die with Parkinson's disease."

As of January 2019, the date of this publication, the causes of Parkinson's disease are not known and there are no treatments that can slow, stop or reverse its progression. There is no known cure. Researchers in a variety of fields are continuing to make slow but deliberate progress with identifying the causes and developing possible cures. What follows is a short, layman's description about what has been discovered and what the goals are as the research continues.

History: What We Know ~ January 2019.

Parkinson's disease is named after the English physician, Dr. James Parkinson (1755-1824), who first described the disease in a publication in 1817 entitled, *An Essay on the Shaking Palsy*. World Parkinson's Day is celebrated every year on April 11th, his birthday. A red tulip is used as a symbolic representation.

Using little more than his skills and his powers of observation, Dr. Parkinson studied six persons who shared similar symptoms which he attributed to this shaking palsy. He incorrectly concluded that the disease was a result of bruising and injury, sometimes from multiple incidents, at the cervical spinal cord. Now we know much which is very different from what Dr. Parkinson described more than 102 years ago.

Years of scientific study and research have taught us that deep within the brain is the circuitry which controls the movements of our bodies. That circuitry is an integrated collection of nerve cell nuclei clusters called the basal ganglia which exist in the forebrain and midbrain inside the cerebral hemispheres. Outside the cerebral hemispheres is another group of basal ganglia nuclei called the substantia nigra.

Post-mortem investigations of the brains of

persons who had a diagnosis of Parkinson's disease have established that the tremors and other physical motor impairments which are characteristic of Parkinson's disease are caused by a loss of dopamine-secreting neurons in the substantia nigra. Dopamine is one organic chemical which serves major important functions within the brain and body.

When the dopamine-secreting neurons are damaged or destroyed the neurotransmission of information is short-circuited, information cannot be passed and physical movements of the body are compromised. It follows that symptoms such as tremor, slowed movement, physical instability and stiffness result. The less dopamine that there is functioning in the brain the greater the manifestation of symptoms, the more difficulty that there is for controlling movement, and the stronger is the grip that Parkinson's has on a person.

Researchers, scientists and members of the medical community generally agree that there are approximately 400,000 dopamine-producing neurons at work within our bodies. A healthy, aging adult loses between 1,000 and 1,500 of these neurons each year. That rate is significantly higher for a person diagnosed with Parkinson's disease. At the time of manifest symptoms and diagnosis that person is estimated to have lost between 275,000 and 325,000 neurons.

Approximately one of every 325 Americans, about one million persons, has been diagnosed with Parkinson's. It is a disease for which

60,000 new cases are diagnosed each year in the United States statistically affecting perhaps 50 percent more men than women.

After Alzheimer's disease, Parkinson's disease is ranked as the second most-common neurodegenerative disorder to which humanity is vulnerable. As described above in the *Overview,* Parkinson's is an age-related disease for which the onset of symptoms and confirmed diagnosis is about age 60.

Research and Results: A Learning Process.

So why, after more than 100 years of an awareness of this shaking palsy, has there been seemingly so little progress in confirming its symptoms and finding a cure? Millions of people throughout the world know that there have been dozens of diseases which have been brought under control or have been eradicated (eliminated forever) because of reasons such as dedicated research, government support and funding, activist movements, medical training, and hospital, laboratory and clinical protocols. Some examples of those diseases are AIDS, malaria, measles, polio and smallpox. All are killer diseases.

But those diseases are infectious diseases. Parkinson's disease is not.

The discovery of vaccines to control and eliminate infectious diseases has been the single greatest factor responsible for reducing their spread. The finest example is that universal immunizations have led to the eradication of smallpox. Other infectious diseases remain a threat.

We citizens of the United States are very fortunate. In this country, immunizations have eliminated almost completely other infectious diseases such as measles, mumps and polio. But HIV, (the virus which causes AIDS), malaria and tuberculosis do not yet have a successful enough vaccine to be considered as effective as those vaccines which have brought the other killer diseases under control.

AIDS is the most recent of these infectious diseases to make an appearance and perhaps easiest for a lay person to understand. In the early 1980's, AIDS, (Acquired Immune Deficiency Syndrome), captured the world's attention when the disease reached pandemic proportions. At that time the causes were unknown and there was no known cure which is true for Parkinson's disease today.

Striking the world community seemingly by surprise, AIDS affected a disproportionate number of men (estimated around 75 percent) than women (estimated around 25 percent). Homosexual men represented more than 70 percent of the men who were infected. Nations and communities invested their resources to identify the causes and find a cure.

Within twenty years the virus HIV, (Human Immunodeficiency Virus), was identified as the cause. HIV attacks the body's immune system and kills by preventing the body from fighting infections and disease. HIV is spread through contact with infected blood, semen, or vaginal fluids, as a result of transfusions from tainted blood, having unprotected sex with someone with HIV, and by sharing drug needles with someone with HIV. HIV can be transmitted from a mother to her baby while pregnant, during birth and while breastfeeding.

But since 2000, monitoring the blood supply, heightened awareness about sharing needles, practicing "safe sex," and testing for HIV, have reduced the spread of AIDS. New infections have fallen by 35 percent.

The discovery and use of drugs which can suppress the HIV virus are keeping more than 15 million AIDS patients alive. Since 2000, AIDS-related deaths have decreased by 40 percent.

Persons with Parkinson's disease, their families, friends and supporters are anxious to see similar such progress. But a degenerative disease which is not caused by a virus and for which a vaccine has no relevance presents enormous challenges.

In the past 100 years, there has been slow but substantial progress investigating, studying and understanding this disease.

In the early 1900's researcher Frederic Lewy identified and described microscopic particles in the brains of persons who had died with Parkinson's disease.

Between 1920 and 1940, further research had

established and proven that, within the brain, the primary cerebral structure that was compromised was the substantia nigra which acts to control movement and other body functions and behaviors.

During the 1950's, researchers identified the chemical dopamine as the neurotransmitter which, when compromised within the brain, results in the manifestation of symptoms. In the mid-1960's, the drug Levodopa (L-dopa) was shown to have an effect on moderating some of the symptoms. It was used widely as treatment.

Twenty years later, surgery, known as deep brain stimulation, demonstrated that the use of electrodes within specific areas of the brain could relieve some of the loss-of-movement symptoms which are associated with Parkinson's disease. Individuals whose symptoms have shown some improvement as a result of medications, but whose symptoms cannot be controlled by them, are candidates who may be helped by this surgical procedure.

After an MRI to identify the specific area of the brain for the surgery, a battery-operated device is implanted. The device generates electrical stimulations which serve to block the abnormal brain signals that are responsible for the symptoms which appear with Parkinson's disease.

Now, in January 2019, the treatment options are only medications and surgery which do no more than manage the symptoms. Improvements with both medications and technology might provide greater help. But still there is no cure.

"Old age hath yet his honor and his toil."

Alfred Tennyson, Poet Laureate, Great Britain and Ireland.

3. THE AGING PROCESS

The Evolution of Our Species.

Had I been Lord Alfred Tennyson's age when he made the statement quoted above, I would have reversed the order of the two words, "honor" and "toil," and said, "Old age hath yet his toil and his honor." It seems to me that the occasions of extraordinary toil when we are younger and at our best to think and work may result in honors later in life for those efforts. Some examples which come to mind are the awards of Nobel Prizes for years of research in science and medicine; Lifetime Achievement Awards for performances in the Arts and Entertainment industry; and, canonization and sainthood for the truly exceptional persons of the Church. In my 67 years of life experiences, I have had far more my share of toil than I have had of honor.

The reality of Parkinson's disease makes a mockery of Lord Tennyson's comment. This age-related degenerative brain disease strikes most persons near or at the time for retirement and the end of a lifetime of toil, privately often as a parent, and frequently professionally often concluding a career. No

33

one who endures its symptoms or suffers the debility would consider it an old age honor.

Somewhere I have read or heard the comment, "we have had nothing to do with our evolution and everything to do with our dissolution." It was made in reference to the transformation within American society where obesity is on the increase, accompanied in direct proportion to the increase in numbers of persons with diabetes, where unhealthy eating habits are epitomized by fast-food consumption, and where exercise consists mainly of moving the mouth and the fingers while using a cell phone.

There have been several revisions of "The Evolution of Man" chart. In one recent revision, the hairy and naked creatures beginning with Ramapithecus and moving progressively through Homo Erectus, Early Homo Sapiens, Neanderthal, Cro-Magnon and finally Modern Homo Sapiens are followed by Neo-Techno Non-Sapien: a bald, obese male wearing a business suit, carrying a box of donuts under his left arm and looking down toward his right side to view the cell phone that he is holding in his right hand. This is not how we humans were meant to evolve.

We have known for some time that 99.9 percent of every human being alive is exactly the same. We are so specialized that even bloodhounds cannot smell the difference between identical twins.

From understanding how Modern Homo Sapiens

evolved from Ramapithecus we know that genetic and physical changes have occurred within our species and probably will continue to occur. Ninety percent of our genes are identical to those of a mouse. Somewhat more than 30 percent of our genes are identical to those of a simple nematode worm! We also have known for some time that every human ailment has some basis in our genes.

On April 14, 2003 the National Human Research Institute (NHRI), the United States Department of Energy (DOE), and the six-nation members of the International Human Genome Sequencing Consortium announced the successful completion of the multibillion-dollar Human Genome Project as planned, under time and under budget. What this Project accomplished was the mapping of our approximately 100,000 genes within our 23 pairs of chromosomes to create a huge genetic blueprint. That blueprint describes the elements and order by which we as human beings have been created. It was done by studying human DNA (Deoxyribonucleic Acid) which is the chemical compound that contains all of the instructions to create and maintain life.

In 1967, Mrs. Rath taught me in tenth grade biology class that DNA is the stuff of my genes, which I inherited from my parents, and that DNA is molecules twisted in two-paired strands, called a double helix. That was discovered and proven by a two-person team of one American and one Englishman who were drinking-buddy researchers in England only 14 years earlier in 1953.

A DNA strand is composed of four chemical units which are called nucleotide bases and which make up our genetic code. The bases are proteins, and the genetic code is a complex order in which those bases are arranged. One gene, assisted by proteins such as hormones and enzymes, makes another protein.

The Human Genome Project confirmed that the protein bases are (A) adenine, (C) cytosine, (G) guanine, and (T) thymine. Bases on opposite DNA strands always are paired in a specific order. The order of these pairings is what creates our genetic code. One estimate is that there are around three and a half billion letters contained within the code.

An ability to read the code and the knowledge of what the code represents give us the means to understand who we are, why we stay healthy, and why we get sick. Soon researchers may be able to identify those genes that may cause not only common illnesses but also such compromising and life-threatening diseases as Alzheimer's, Parkinson's, cancer, diabetes and heart disease. Eight genes have been linked to Alzheimer's disease.

Only about one to two percent of persons diagnosed with Parkinson's disease have the genes which result in the disease. The majority of others who are vulnerable to Parkinson's carry linked or supplemental genes which reflect the person's vulnerability because of genetic predisposition but which do not determine that that the disease actually will develop.

Presently, it is assumed that killer diseases such as cancer are caused by compromises in the interaction within our genes and the possible combination of those interactions and the effects of our environment. The work that has been accomplished by all those who supported the Human Genome Project should give us the possibility, even the promise, of a future ability to cure these diseases.

Life Expectancy.

Historically, life expectancy has been increasing for most people in most parts of the world. We all age differently. Factors which influence life expectancy are genetic makeup, sex, location, and the political, social, economic and environmental conditions where we live.

Prehistoric man (both sexes) lived to an average age between 20 and 35 years. Medieval Europeans and 18th century Eurasians averaged between 30 and 40 years. Throughout the world, the average life expectancy in 1900 was between 35 and 40 years; in 1950 it was between 45 and 50 years; and, in 2000 it was between 65 and 70 years.

Even though the Human Genome Project may be considered the greatest human scientific achievement ever by opening the door for our present and future generations to understand how we are made, what makes us function, and what may cause us to die, we still will look to our generational lineage for what may be a better indication of our longevity. How long did our parents, our grandparents and our great-grandparents live, and what were the causes for their deaths? Presently, genetic research gives us only an indication of our susceptibility to illness and disease but no confirmation that the vulnerability is a certainty. With respect to Parkinson's disease, approximately 15 to 25 percent of persons who have or had the disease have family members who share or shared it.

Next, among humans worldwide, female life expectancy is measurably higher than that for males. There are many reasons why this is true. Recall, as described earlier in the narrative, how we as a species have evolved. In most other animal species, excluding birds, with which we share more than 95 percent of our genes, males have higher mortality than females. In 2007, Professor John Santrock determined that females have been shown to have a greater resistance to infections, illnesses and certain degenerative diseases.

Males tend to have more physical, labor-intensive, and dangerous occupations, such as military service, industry, transportation, shipping and farming. Their numbers also lead those of females in life-threatening habits, such as smoking, alcohol consumption and substance abuse, as well as the more life-threatening hobbies such race-car driving, mountaineering, white-water rafting and other extreme sports.

Where we live is a third indicator of longevity. People who live in countries in the developed world live, on average, longer than people in the developing world. Those countries where the availability and quality of universal health care for its citizens are a national priority have a high life expectancy ranking. This is especially true in those countries with a low infant mortality rate.

The World Health Organization has published statistics which indicate that life expectancy is the longest (between 81 and 84 years) for someone living in Europe or in Asia (Japan, South Korea and Singapore). It is the lowest (between 50 and 60 years) for persons living in 25 nations in Africa where ongoing wars and HIV infections are decimating the population.

In the United States, U.S. Federal government data as of December 2007 indicate that women at age 65 can expect to live to age 87, and men at age 65 can expect to live to age 84.

As We Age.

From studying and analyzing the fossil evidence of our evolution from Ramapithecus to Modern Homo Sapiens and from viewing computer-generated images using that information of our evolution from 100,000 to 10,000 years ago, the human population has become smaller. Evidence shows that we have evolved with slighter bone structure, lighter physical color and more diverse and distinctive facial features. Our jaws have become smaller and our teeth larger and more crowded within our mouths.

We know that the aging process affects every part of our bodies which go through a variety of changes as we age. We shrink as we age as a result of the compression of the discs which compose our spines.

Over time, even with a regular routine of aerobic exercise, our hearts, as a muscle, become less efficient. It pumps with less force causing our cells which use oxygen to absorb less. Before age 40 almost everyone loses some degree of aerobic capacity.

Other muscles also become weaker and shrink in size and density. Between the ages of 50 and 70 we lose an average of 25 percent of our muscle mass and capacity.

Our bones become weaker and shrink in size and density. This is especially true for women at menopause when their bones may lose 10 to 20 percent of their density. Over time, more than 50 percent of women age 50 and older will suffer an injury resulting in a broken bone.

Our skin, blood vessels and tissues slowly lose their elasticity. We may bruise more easily and see the evidence of bruising as discolorations on our skin.

Our eyes become affected. Beginning about age 40, the lenses of our eyes become more rigid. Their muscle fibers decline. The ability to focus easily on objects both near and far becomes compromised. Many seniors require glasses to read or see distinctly. Cataracts, floaters and other eye-related problems develop. Between the ages of 45 and 55 the rates of macular degeneration and glaucoma, which can lead to blindness, double.

At about the same time, many seniors experience a diminished ability to hear well as a result of overall or range-specific hearing loss. They require the use of hearing aids to restore good and well-balanced hearing. Hearing loss also affects a person's equilibrium and, accordingly, his sense of balance and controlled movement.

Men who still are student-age may begin to lose their hair as a result of natural hormones which control and reduce hair follicles. As they age, more men lose some or all of their hair. What hair a person of either sex may retain begins to turn various shades of gray and white around age 50.

Mentally, our memory, alertness and situational awareness may diminish and become less reliable. Overall, our metabolism and many bodily functions slow down. Beginning at about age 40, the human brain starts to lose about five percent of its volume approximately every 10 years.

Finally, as we age we become vulnerable to a variety of age-related health problems which are a result of our genetics, our environment, and our lifestyles, behaviors and habits. More than 90 percent of diseases are caused or complicated by stress.

Heart disease is the number-one killer striking people with chronically high blood pressure and cholesterol. Because these factors do not manifest any symptoms, heart attacks and strokes are the earliest and first indications of serious problems.

Cancer is the number-two killer and results from a variety of causes such as genetics, environment, and substance abuse. Many types of cancer are treatable and survivable if detected early through medical screenings. As if weren't bad enough that smoking has been demonstrated to cause cancer, second-hand smoke contains more than 4,000 chemicals including more than 40 cancer-causing compounds. Second-hand smoke contains twice as much tar and nicotine per unit volume as does smoke inhaled from a cigarette, three times as much cancer-causing benzopyrene, and five times as much carbon monoxide. Secondary smoke from pipes and cigars is equally as harmful.

Respiratory disease is the number-three killer. Persons with asthma, chronic bronchitis and emphysema are at greater risk for pneumonia and other lung infections. For example, COPD (Chronic Obstructive Pulmonary Disease) is a progressively debilitating disease, with symptoms such as coughing and wheezing, which results after the airways to the lungs have been damaged and the ability to breathe becomes more difficult as the disease worsens.

Almost 50 percent of seniors over age 65 suffer from arthritis, a painful condition of the joints, which may restrict mobility and activity and diminish a person's quality of life.

Alzheimer's disease affects approximately one of every nine persons age 65 or older. Like Parkinson's disease, it is a chronic neurodegenerative disease that, also like Parkinson's, starts slowly and worsens over time. Manifest systems include short-term memory loss, disorientation, difficulty communicating and personality changes such as mood swings. The condition leads to death usually within ten years after diagnosis.

There are other challenges which affect seniors as they age. They may have a medical basis which causes injury or illness as a result of behavioral issues. Osteoporosis and osteo-arthritis can lead to falls and broken bones. Depression can lead to substance abuse. Obesity can lead to diabetes and cardio-pulmonary disease.

As was written earlier in the narrative, "we have evolved to die." Dying and death often are accompanied with some measure of sadness. As we age, we strive for a happy and balanced life and to become better men and women. It should be important and helpful for us to know the natural biological order of our existence. Understanding that should be meaningful for

us to be able to recognize, know and confront
those diseases, illnesses and events which are
beyond our control and which may challenge us
as we age. I believe that we should do so with
a sense of purpose, patience and peace.

"Everyone needs to be proactive and know the various warning signs of disease. Early detection and research to make detection easier at earlier stages, along with the treatments needs, still is a must."

Dennis Franz, American actor.

4. SIGNS AND SYMPTOMS

Many people know from reading history and from viewing documentaries about war that the service member in combat who is fighting a battle or who is closest to the battlefield is the most accurate and reliable source for information about what is happening or what has happened. As a veteran, I know this to be true. I have the same sense of awareness for the signs and symptoms of Parkinson's disease. The individual himself or his spouse, companion with whom he may be living, children, other close family members, neighbors and coworkers who are in frequent contact with someone usually are the first to detect the signs and symptoms. Together they may initiate the process which will lead to a diagnosis. A confirmed diagnosis of Parkinson's disease starts the course of action for specific care, medications, support, therapy and the management of manifest symptoms.

Stages.

Within the scientific and medical communities, the word, "epidemiology" refers to the identification and description of the elements which characterize health-related problems as they are discovered and progress over time, and the use of that information to manage and control those health problems. Almost always there is a natural history disease timeline associated with specific diseases. For example, the "Period of Susceptibility" and the "Period of Exposure" begin the timeline for infectious diseases. The "Incidents of Physical Changes" and "Onset of Symptoms" begin the timeline for neurodegenerative diseases such as Alzheimer's disease and Parkinson's disease. Timelines make it easier to recognize, treat, evaluate, manage and control disease. Generally, within the reference literature and the medical community, there are five "Stages" which describe Parkinson's disease.

Stage One describes mild symptoms such as tremor affecting either the left or right side of the body only (unilateral) and also may include symptoms affecting the back and neck. There may be obvious changes in a person's posture and facial expressions. Usually the symptoms at this stage do not affect a person's ability to live alone, act routinely and maintain his lifestyle.

Stage Two describes mild symptoms affecting both sides of the body (bilateral) and also may include problems associated with posture and balance. In this stage the initial symptoms are more manifest and difficult to control. A person may find it challenging to fasten a button, use a zipper, stand from a seated position, walk between rooms or address and write a card or letter. It becomes somewhat harder for a person to continue to live alone and to maintain his daily routine and lifestyle. In these early Stages One and Two, the manifestation of symptoms may change during the day appearing as mild or severe or disappear entirely.

Stage Three describes mid-term Parkinson's when a person who still may be independent has problems reading, writing, eating, bathing, dressing and communicating. Movement is slowed considerably and a greater loss of balance may result in falls.

Stage Four describes early disability Parkinson's when a person loses his independence, usually can no longer live alone, and requires help standing, walking, reading, writing, eating, bathing and dressing. His routine has become more dependent and his lifestyle has slowed significantly.

Stage Five describes late-term Parkinson's when the disease has seized control of a person's body and compromised his physical and mental abilities. Persons at this stage no longer are able to care for themselves, require help standing and moving, usually require the use of a wheelchair for mobility, may be institutionalized for health and safety reasons, and are most vulnerable to increased challenges with their health and body functions.

The signs and symptoms of Parkinson's disease vary with every person. Not everyone with Parkinson's will experience all of the most-common symptoms in each of the stages. Also, the degree or intensity with which the symptoms manifest themselves can vary significantly. Many factors such as a person's age, general health, physical and mental condition, medications, diet, lifestyle and environment have an influence. Symptoms may be more pronounced and exacerbated when a person is ill, dehydrated, sleep deprived, stressed, has experienced recent surgery or changes to prescribed medications.

Core Motor Symptoms.

The majority of persons who have received a diagnosis for Parkinson's disease and those persons who are closest in relationship to them usually first notice the onset of the disease in one or more of the four core motor symptoms. Those symptoms are: Bradykinesia, tremor, rigidity and postural instability. These symptoms are usually asymmetric.

Bradykinesia is the slowness of voluntary movement and speech. Tremor is the involuntary movement of a body part such as the hand, arm, foot or leg. Frequently it is the most recognizable symptom starting at the onset of

48

Parkinson's. Rigidity is the physical stiffness or lack of flexibility of limbs and other body parts as a result of continuous involuntary muscle contractions. Postural instability is the varying physical disorientation of the torso which may lean forward or to either side, the reduced movement or natural swing of either or both arms during movement, and the slowed and shuffled gait when walking. Studies have shown that the process of dopamine loss may begin as early as five years prior to the development of motor symptoms

Associated Physical Symptoms: The Senses.

All of the five primary senses, (sight, taste, smell, touch and hearing) with which a person's basic functioning and awareness of his environment are established, maintained, evaluated, and controlled are affected by Parkinson's disease. Some effects are debilitating; others are life-threatening.

Sight is the ability to perceive objects through the use of our eyes. Sight may be affected in several ways. The slowness associated with motor movement also occurs in the eyes. The frequency or rate at which a person blinks may slow. When it does, a dry eye condition may result because the normal rate of tearing, which provides moisture to the eyes, slows. A person may have difficulty opening his eyes or his eyes may be partially or fully closed. This condition is caused sometimes by the medications used to treat Parkinson's disease. Changes to the normal routine of tearing also may cause irritation at the eye surface. A person may have difficulty viewing objects, focusing on objects or staring at them. Difficulty with eye convergence may result in eye strain, blurred vision or double vision. Some persons who are able to see relatively clearly during the day may have trouble seeing at night or in the dark.

Taste is the ability to determine the flavor of food or other substances which enter the mouth and react with the tongue and taste receptors within the mouth. There is a heightened awareness for foods which are sweet, sour, salty or bitter. Parkinson's disease may affect the sense of taste most directly by affecting a person's sense of smell and the ability to detect flavor. Certain tastes are compromised by the influence of various prescribed drugs. Persons with difficulty swallowing become detached from recognizing and appreciating the taste of foods which they may be struggling to swallow. Also, persons with general apathy or depression brought on by Parkinson's disease may lose interest in eating and may consider their food to be bland.

Smell is the ability to detect and distinguish odors and aromas in our environment. This is accomplished by the olfactory bulb which is the part of the brain that transmits smell signals from sensory neurons in the nose. When the transmission circuitry for these neurons within the brain are compromised by the degenerative effects of Parkinson's disease then a person's sense of smell is compromised. The gradual loss of the sense of smell is a more common early symptom for the onset of Parkinson's disease.

Touch is the sense of feeling and recognizing something with the use of our hands. The skin on our hands uses nerve endings to create the sense of touch. When a person experiences sensations such as pain, heat, cold or feels things that are soft, sticky or sharp, the bottom layer of his skin, called the dermis, sends messages to the brain about the sensation. Through the sense of touch we are able to recognize temperatures, feel discomfort or pain and distinguish many physical characteristics of other human beings and inanimate objects. We use our hands in most of the activities which we do during the day: tending to personal hygiene, dressing, eating, working, communicating, exercising, making contact and interacting with other people. Because Parkinson's disease affects movement and the muscles which enable movement, the hands of people with Parkinson's often become stiffer, and the fingers less flexible. At later stages, the fingers may be curled and locked into fists which makes it difficult, if not impossible, to initiate or complete the tasks associated with a person's daily activities.

Hearing is the ability to recognize and identify sounds through the use of our ears. In Chapter 3, "The Aging Process," there is a short statement about any hearing loss as a natural, age-related condition. The sensory organ of hearing is called the cochlea. It is located within the inner ear. The cochlea is affected by Parkinson's disease because it is protected by the chemical dopamine from noise exposure. The loss of dopamine cells, which characterizes Parkinson's disease, may damage the cochlea and result in a hearing loss.

Accompanying Mental or Emotional Symptoms.

For most persons with Parkinson's disease the *"Core Motor Symptoms"* and the *"Associated Physical Symptoms"* precede any *"Accompanying Mental or Emotional Symptoms."* On average, after the onset of symptoms and a confirmed diagnosis for Parkinson's disease, a person may experience problems with his autonomic system (body temperature, blood pressure, heart rate, respiration rate, digestion and more), disposition and temperament, sleep and cognitive decline. All of the symptoms, most notably cognitive decline, greatly increase the extent of a person's disability.

Cognitive disturbances and decline may be observed earlier; however, in the early stages this decline may be a result of other causes such as age-related dementia or Alzheimer's disease. Problems with a person's memory usually do not occur in the early stages. As Parkinson's disease advances so does the incidence of dementia. With respect to the dementia that is characteristic of Alzheimer's disease, a person with Alzheimer's has lost entirely certain information. However, most persons with Parkinson's disease usually experiences only difficulty retrieving and communicating information. There also may be problems related to a person's attention, focus and concentration.

Sleep disturbances may be characterized by a sense of feeling tired and sleepy during the day, an inability to fall asleep at night, difficulty while sleeping and difficulty staying asleep. Waking early is common.

Depression is an emotional symptom present within more than 35 and close to 50 percent of persons with Parkinson's disease. It is one of the most common neuropsychiatric conditions found in persons with Parkinson's. Studies indicate that the depression associated with Parkinson's is a result of the disease itself since Parkinson's affects many areas of the brain that control a person's mood. The diminished levels of dopamine in the brain is more responsible for depression than are the person's sentiments about his disability.

Psychotic symptoms, such as paranoia, delusions and hallucinations, are common. Most hallucinations are visual, usually involve seeing things which are not there, such as persons or pets very familiar to the person and are non-threatening. Research indicates that a person's hallucinations may be the result of drug therapy focused on the dopamine levels in the brain. Chemical and physical changes resulting from this type of therapy may be responsible for the hallucinations which usually do not occur until the late stages of the disease.

Because these and other symptoms occur gradually over several years it is difficult to diagnose Parkinson's disease. No two persons have the same set of symptoms which have occurred at the same time of life with the same intensity, duration and responses to medication, therapy and lifestyle changes. I have read the comment, "when you have seen one Parkinson's patient, you have seen one Parkinson's patient." Therefore, at the earliest time when symptoms manifest themselves to someone, his family, his closest friends or coworkers it is essential to seek a professional diagnosis in order to manage and control the progression of this disease.

"Doctors are our partners, and they need all the assistance we can give them to be sure we get the right diagnosis."

Ann Richards, Former Governor of Texas.

5. THE DIAGNOSIS

For eight years between 2004 and 2012 I served as a volunteer test subject at the University of Texas Medical Branch (UTMB) in Galveston, Texas. The University had access to my medical records which included my annual physicals beginning in 1969 as a Cadet at West Point through my retirement at NASA's Johnson Space Center in 2011. I participated in a variety of studies related to healthy aging because the data within those medical records showed that for almost 42 years my physiological statistics had varied only slightly. My weight moved between 145 and 149 pounds; my blood pressure averaged 110 / 65 (unless I had been driving on the Houston highways); my resting heart rate was usually 50 beats per minute.

During the lengthy interviews and screenings with the medical doctors, the research study principal investigators and their technical assistants, and the nursing staff I often heard them say that everything I said or wrote was extremely important to their study. The sentiment was that my personal data and statistics gave the research team the information necessary to apply the parameters from the design the study to me for such considerations as length, procedures, diet, exercise, rest and medications based upon my reported and documented health status.

The symptoms of Parkinson's disease occur gradually over several years. In its early stages, Parkinson's is not easy to diagnose. There is no measurable indicator such as a blood test, a brain scan or an ElectroEncephaloGram (EEG) to confirm that there is some biological state or condition which causes Parkinson's disease.

Among the early onset symptoms, tremor and problems associated with posture and balance are those which a person and the people closest to him notice first. These serious core motor symptoms are a disconcerting surprise, blatantly obvious and seemingly occurring without any precondition illness or injury. Very quickly a person will ask his spouse, family member, friend or coworker something such as "Have you ever noticed my left hand shaking?" or "Do I look as if I'm bent over or standing crooked?"

From having spoken with many persons whose family members or friends had been diagnosed with Parkinson's disease I learned that they usually were not the first to ask about what they had observed as a physical abnormality. Sympathetic to this, the most direct question someone may have asked was, "Are you feeling alright?" or "Is everything OK with you?" The discussion which ensued usually resulted in the decision to make an appointment with the person's family medical doctor or health care provider.

Without any determinant indicator to confirm a diagnosis for Parkinson's disease, the diagnosis usually is the result of the work of two doctors: the person's family medical doctor or health care provider and a neurologist. It is a diagnosis which takes time to confirm.

At the initial appointment, the doctor will listen to his patient's complaints, observe at least one of the early onset symptoms, review his family medical history and conduct a complete medical examination. Then, if after having ruled out other possible reasons for the condition such as illness, injury or medication, the doctor may suspect Parkinson's disease as the cause, it is usual for him to refer his patient to a neurologist. It is very important that the neurologist is someone who is very familiar and has experience with Parkinson's disease.

A neurologist is a doctor who is trained to diagnose and treat problems related to the brain and nervous system. The examination by the neurologist contains all of the procedures as those conducted by the family doctor and more. It is a far more extensive and lengthy examination usually extending over several visits. Normally two of the four main symptoms must be present over a period of time for a neurologist to confirm a diagnosis for Parkinson's disease.

After a discussion about the length of experience and the character of the symptoms the neurologist will investigate the patient's family history of any neurological diseases. He also will seek an understanding of the patient's environment and lifestyle with respect to work history and conditions such as any exposure to toxins, social habits such as the use of drugs and alcohol, and history of illnesses, injuries, trauma and hospitalizations.

Consistent with the signs and symptoms which appear in the stages of Parkinson's disease and which were described in the previous chapter, the neurologist may conduct a series of additional tests. These tests serve to observe and evaluate the patient's speech, vision and focus, reflexes and reactions to stimulation, balance, coordination and muscle strength. For patients who are manifesting symptoms indicative of the early stages of Parkinson's, many of these tests may be repeated after two or more weeks for a period of six to eight weeks. The neurologist also may include brain imaging to help with his diagnosis.

If the neurologist suspects Parkinson's disease as the cause he may prescribe one of several Parkinson's-related medications such as carbidopa-levodopa to be taken for several weeks or a few months. Parkinson's patients take a number of a variety of medications to manage their symptoms. The medications will substitute for or increase dopamine, the chemical in the brain which is responsible for controlling signals for physical movement.

The purpose is to determine if and to what degree the symptoms are affected by the medication. If the patient reports significant improvement, such as less frequent or milder tremor or more stability while walking, then the neurologist usually will confirm a diagnosis for Parkinson's disease. The most accurate diagnosis is obtained by medical doctors and clinic specialists using standard diagnostic criteria and long-term observation. More than 80 percent of the diagnoses for Parkinson's disease were confirmed and proven accurate.

The good news is that a diagnosis is not a death sentence. Parkinson's is not a killer disease. The other-than-good news is that the symptoms of Parkinson's disease will continue and worsen over time. The cause is unknown.

"Genetics loads the gun and the environment pulls the trigger."

Michael J. Fox with David Letterman, 2015.

6.   POSSIBLE CAUSES

Many people who may be aware of the stories about the hundreds of famous men and women with Parkinson's disease, such as the entertainers Michael J. Fox and Linda Ronstadt, do not know what causes the disease or that there is no cure for it. More surprisingly is the fact that now, in 2019, the scientific and medical communities also do not know the causes but do know that there is no cure. Today, researchers at prestigious institutions such as the National Institutes of Health (NIH) and The National Institute of Environmental Health Sciences (NIEHS) believe that the onset of Parkinson's disease is the result of a combination of genetic and environmental factors much like what Michael J. Fox said to David Letterman in 2015.

World War II began in September 1939 with Germans and Poles fighting each other riding on horseback and firing single-shot rifles. It ended in August 1945 after two atomic bombs were dropped on Japan. How could there be such a dramatic difference in warfare in only six years yet no such dramatic difference *At War with Parkinson's Disease* after more than 100 years of research involving thousands of case studies and hundreds of millions of dollars?

Part, if not most, of the answer may be the complexity of the disease, its foundations within the brain and its effect on multiple sensory systems which make the body function. Because Parkinson's is an age-related degenerative disease usually occurring in persons age 60 and older there are not many years with which to study someone by long-term observations and testing. A baseline history for a study describing symptoms, their origins and a person's physical, mental and emotional status cannot be established because it is not possible to know when the symptoms first started, only when they began to manifest themselves.

Different symptoms manifest themselves at different times, for different durations and at different levels of severity. Symptoms may come and go or not appear at all during the day.

Each person's prior medical history and health status at the time of manifest symptoms is different so that research studies requiring standardizations are almost impossible to correlate. Time is needed to evaluate and understand the long-term influence of various medications and differing dosages as well as associated therapies and surgeries which require recovery time after each new procedure.

Given the fact that the cause or causes are

unknown, the volume of research studies which have been conducted for more than 100 years suggest that there are at least five risk factors which may influence and lead to a diagnosis for Parkinson's disease. Those factors are: age, genetics, occupation and occupational hazards, medical events and lifestyle. The remainder of this chapter describes the influence of these factors.

Age.

Several times throughout the narrative the statement appears that Parkinson's disease affects predominantly the elderly. It is the greatest risk factor for the development and advancement of this disease. The average age for the onset is 60 affecting approximately one percent of the population. Parkinson's may affect persons much younger. But only about 15 percent of the cases that confirmed diagnoses for Parkinson's disease have been for individuals who were 40 years old or younger. Studies have shown that the most significant factor contributing to the progression of Parkinson's disease is advancing age and the body's associated natural decline and debilitation, most importantly neurodegeneration.

Genetics.

Since there is not yet a single determinant for the cause of Parkinson's disease, such as the certainty that the Plasmodium parasite causes Malaria and the Variola virus causes

Small Pox, most researchers now believe that the onset of Parkinson's is due to a combination of genetic and environmental factors.

In my family, both my mother Dorothy and her sister Katherine, senior to her by four years, received a confirmed diagnosis for Parkinson's disease. At the time of diagnosis my mother was 77; her sister was 70. Within our extended family there never has been anyone else with this disease.

Some researchers believe that if there are three or more members of a family who have received a confirmed diagnosis for Parkinson's disease at any age then genetics may be the cause or a contributing cause. One or more genes may be responsible.

Earlier in this narrative at Chapter 3, "The Aging Process," is a description of the work by the National Human Genome Research Institute (NHGRI), the United States Department of Energy (DOE), and the six-nation members of the International Human Genome Sequencing Consortium which completed the Human Genome Project in April 2013. That Project successfully mapped the approximately 100,000 genes within our 23 pairs of chromosomes to create a human genetic blueprint.

But before then, in 1997, researchers at NHGRI studied one extended family from Italy in which they knew that several cases of Parkinson's disease had been inherited from parent to child. The research team was able to identify the gene which caused the family's inherited Parkinson's disease. That gene became one small part of the huge genetic code and was identified for a protein called alpha-synuclein.

Further research using the brains from persons who have died with Parkinson's disease established that this alpha-synuclein protein was present in large amounts. Because of the work by NHGRI and others, the research community now knows that the protein alpha-synuclein is dominant in persons with Parkinson's disease. It is the alpha-synuclein proteins in the brain which clump together and which cause the death of dopamine-producing cells that results in Parkinson's disease. The exact process by which this happens continues to be studied.

Beyond the protein alpha-synuclein, the NHGRI team also has identified seven genes that cause some form of Parkinson's disease and may be responsible for early-onset Parkinson's.

Researchers continue to learn why some persons with a genetic marker for Parkinson's disease develop symptoms and die with Parkinson's, and why others with the seemingly identical genetic predisposition live full lives unburdened by the disease. This is the primary reason why many professionals in the research, scientific and medical communities believe that there are environmental and life-experience factors which also contribute to the onset of Parkinson's. They may pull the trigger.

The more that research teams such as NHGRI learn about genetics the more we recognize how complex and complicated the human body and brain are, and how truly mysterious and remarkable has been our evolution. Babies born this year in 2019 share more than 30 percent of their genetic DNA with those of a simple nematode worm and 96 percent of their DNA with those of a chimpanzee.

Gender.

As a risk factor, gender is a key component. Over the past 20 years, almost all research studies conducted throughout the world which have investigated gender as a contributing factor for Parkinson's disease have demonstrated that there is a greater incidence among men than among women. The relative risk is approximately 1.5 times greater for men than for women. A number of studies also have reported sex differences in the severity of symptoms between males and females with Parkinson's disease, and that symptoms start to appear at an earlier age for men than for women. The reasons for these findings are not known conclusively; however, there are several probable contributing factors.

One possible factor which may protect women is that their production of estrogen may have a neuroprotective effect. Studies have demonstrated that there is a beneficial regulatory influence of estrogen on the dopaminergic system, which may validate the possible protective effects of estrogen with respect to Parkinson's disease.

There are other reasons which may explain the differences between men and women and their susceptibility for Parkinson's. They include occupational hazards with work dominated by men such as farming, industrial labor and the military; a higher rate of head trauma from work- or recreational-related activities such as sports and hobbies; and, differences in lifestyles.

Occupation and Occupational Hazards.

There have been a variety of numerous studies which have investigated the possibility that certain occupations and their associated hazards may be environmental risk factors for the onset of Parkinson's disease. These studies have been difficult to design, conduct and evaluate, and the results often have been inconclusive or inconsistent with the results of similar studies.

The occupational environments which have dominated the studies include farming, industry and the military where persons may have been exposed to toxins such as pesticides, chemicals, defoliants and gases. Members of the military may have a compound occupational risk factor given the potential for head injuries from training, routine duty and combat-related trauma. Of all the chemical exposures that have been linked to Parkinson's disease, pesticides have been reported the most frequently and the most consistently.

Farming.

Farming and the exposure of farmers, farm hands and their families to pesticides is an exceptionally difficult occupation to study as an environmental risk factor for the onset of Parkinson's disease. This is true for a variety of reasons.

First, it is only after a farmer, farm hand or member of their families had obtained a diagnosis for Parkinson's that researchers are able to study the symptoms and attempt to evaluate his exposure. Next, there is the significant difficulty creating a population baseline or comparative basis for study. Is it possible to create a valid and reliable regression model for a given population? What factors are important and relevant, and can these factors be quantified? How long had the person been living in a farm community and farming? Is there a distinction among dairy, animal and crop farmers, farm hands and their families? To what specific pesticides or combination of pesticides had he been exposed? What was the length of each exposure? What were the environmental conditions (weather, temperature, wind, precipitation) during the exposure? What was the person's age, physical condition and health? Finally, no farmer or farm hand who started work as a teenager or in his early 20's and who worked for 20 or 30 years or more before the onset of symptoms would know this information. Neither would any member of his family. Surveys which try to qualify and quantify such issues as these often are incomplete, imprecise and possibly inaccurate. Therefore, only a generalized window describing non-quantified possible factors for risk could be used to design a survey and profile for comparison with others from the farming community.

Pesticides include a large number of different chemical compounds which usually are grouped into categories such as fumigants, fungicides, herbicides, insecticides and rodenticides. Their uses are quite varied. Over time, because of a heightened awareness of the toxicity of certain chemical compounds which are used in pesticides and the advances in technology used to manufacture them, the chemicals have changed substantially.

Given this, an investigation conducted in Washington state by researchers from the University of Washington and a Washington state health care system and published in 2005 by the *Journal of the American Medical Association* concluded that "our findings do not provide strong support for the hypothesis that pesticide exposure is a risk factor for Parkinson's disease."

Three years later, another investigation conducted by BioMed Neurology and published in 2008 came to an entirely different conclusion. It stated that "in a study conducted in samples of unrelated individuals, pesticides such as insecticides and herbicides significantly increased the risk of Parkinson's disease."

After another six years, an article in *Scientific American*, published in 2014, stated that "farmers are more prone to Parkinson's than the general population. . .and pesticides could be to blame. Over a decade of evidence shows a clear association between pesticide exposure and a higher risk for Parkinson's disease." The differences among the study designs which were used makes it problematic to compare results.

I am reminded of the question asked jokingly, "What are the three types of lies?" and the answer, "Lies, dam*ed lies and statistics."

Moving on with some good news: Most people who are exposed to pesticides do not go on to become symptomatic and develop Parkinson's disease.

Still the research continues.

Similar to farming, industrial occupations present as difficult an environment to quantify and to study in order to determine what hazards exist, if any, which may present a risk for the onset of Parkinson's disease. However, unlike in farm communities, where farmers and their families work and live at the same location, industrial workers do not live with their families where they work.

Industry.

As with pesticides, humans routinely are exposed to industrial toxicants either at work, elsewhere in the environment or from the use of common household products. There have been numerous studies to determine if a person's exposure to contaminants such as metals, solvents and gases is a risk factor for the onset of Parkinson's disease.

Researchers have confirmed that some symptoms consistent with the onset of Parkinson's disease have occurred in individuals who were exposed to high levels of toxic substances such as carbon disulfide and carbon monoxide, neurotoxic metals such as lead and manganese and organophosphate pesticides such as those discussed previously. In such cases, researchers have extended and expanded their studies to investigate whether or not any exposure to these environmental toxins result in only mimicking some of the symptoms of Parkinson's disease or actually present a confirmed risk for the onset of the disease.

The Military.

Over the years, several studies have concluded that head trauma is a risk factor for neurodegenerative disorders. One of the reasons for this conclusion is that some of the studies which examined brains cells from under a microscope showed that trauma to the head could cause proteins to clump together. Protein clumps are characteristic of Parkinson's disease. As the clumps build and thicken they can cause cell membranes to burst resulting in a loss of brain cells.

No one disputes the fact that the military is a very dangerous profession. As of the date of the publication of this narrative, the United States and its allies have been waging the Global War on Terror for 17 years. Casualties for the United States alone, that is, those not including any from a dozen or more Allied supporters, are more than 7,000 U.S. military killed and more than 50,000 U.S. military wounded. Perhaps as many as one in five of those wounded casualties has suffered head trauma or a Traumatic Brain Injury (TBI) as a result of combat from direct fire, indirect fire, Improvised Explosive Devices (IED's), suicide bombings, other forms of terrorist attacks, crashes and accidents.

Only two years ago, in March 2017, the Clinical Journal of the American College of Neurology published in *Neurology* a case-controlled study entitled, "Head Injury and risk for Parkinson's disease." The researchers studied 1,705 patients with confirmed diagnoses for Parkinson's disease from within 10 neurologic centers in Denmark during the years 1996 – 2009. These researchers concluded that, "The results do not support the hypothesis that head injury increases the risk for Parkinson's disease."

Then, just 13 months later, the same journal, *Neurology*, published a study which contradicted that finding and concluded instead that Traumatic Brain Injury (TBI) is associated with an increased risk of Parkinson's disease. The Centers for Disease Control (CDC) defines "Traumatic Brain Injury" as a "disruption in the normal function of the brain that can be caused by a bump, blow, or jolt to the head, or penetrating head injury."

In that study, published in April 2018, researchers examined the medical records of 325,870 veterans. Approximately half of these veterans had a record of a mild, moderate or severe traumatic brain injury. (The terms "mild," "moderate," and "severe" were defined in the study as follows: "Mild" was a loss of consciousness for less than 30 minutes and memory loss for less than 24 hours. "Moderate" to "Severe" were defined as loss of consciousness for more than 30 minutes and memory loss for more than 24 hours.)

When the study began, none of the veterans had received a confirmed diagnosis for Parkinson's disease. But, within 12 years, there were 1,462 of these veterans who did receive a confirmed diagnosis for Parkinson's, 949 of whom also had a confirmed diagnosis for traumatic brain injury.

After the researchers refined the results by adjusting for age, prior and existing medical conditions and other discriminating factors, they concluded that a "mild TBI" increases the risk for Parkinson's disease by 56 percent and that a "moderate to severe TBI" increases the risk by 83 percent.

Concluding here with some more good news: of the 325,870 veterans who supported this wide study only less than one percent of them received a confirmed diagnosis for Parkinson's disease even if they had experienced a traumatic brain injury.

Medical Events.

Certain prior medical events of a serious nature, such as head trauma, viruses, other illnesses, inflammations and tumors, would seem to be potential risk factors for the onset of Parkinson's disease. However, with the exception of head trauma which was described above and specific viruses, the literature suggests that the opposite is true. A person's debilitation as a result of the effects of Parkinson's disease may be the cause for vulnerability to more serious illnesses, tumors and cancers as he lives and ages with the disease.

The most serious virus for which research suggests a link to the onset of Parkinson's disease is the HIV virus which causes AIDS. This virus attacks and destroys the peripheral immune system and very quickly enters the brain. Within about two weeks after infection, the brain and central nervous system are damaged, neurons are compromised and motor functions are impaired. In the brain, the HIV virus has been demonstrated to infect astrocytes which anchor neurons to their blood supply permitting specific substances to pass between the blood and the brain, and to infect microglia which ingest dead tissue and fight threats. The ability of the brain to generate dopamine and the loss of dopamine in the brain results in the onset of Parkinson's disease.

Other viruses also may enter the brain, especially those associated with illnesses that are accompanied by very high fever and inflammation, and may compromise the brain's ability to communicate neurologically.

Lifestyles.

Addiction is a medical disorder that affects the brain and changes behavior. The use and abuse of alcohol, nicotine, prescription and illegal drugs cost Americans more than $700 billion a year in health care costs, lost productivity, crime and social disruptions.

Alcohol and drugs affect the way a person feels by altering the chemicals in the brain, the most complex of all the organs in the human body. The feel-good sensations result from alcohol- or drug-induced changes to brain circuits that affect reward, stress, and self-control. The use and abuse of alcohol and drugs results in negative physiological effects such as altered brain chemistry, health problems, infections, injuries, accidents, disability and death.

Most of the pleasurable effects of illegal drug use are believed to result from the release of high levels of the neurotransmitter dopamine. Within the body, dopamine is the chemical associated with motivation, the feeling of pleasure, and motor function. Drugs, such as cocaine and methamphetamine, which increase the release of dopamine, may harm the nerve terminals within the brain. The inability of dopamine to function in the brain and the loss of dopamine cells are factors which affect motor functions and which lead to the onset of Parkinson's disease.

Chronic cocaine abusers have been found to have decreased levels of dopamine. A research investigation published by the National Institutes of Health in January 2012 studied a California-based population of individuals at least 30 years of age who had been hospitalized for the use / abuse of the drug methamphetamine. The group was studied for a period of 16 years. Data from the research indicated that methamphetamine users have an above-normal risk for developing Parkinson's disease.

Beyond being significantly drunk or high, persons in such states may up the ante for irresponsibility. They may share infected needles while doing drugs and may engage in unprotected sex. In those cases, exposure to the HIV virus and its ability to infect the brain, disrupt or block the neurotransmission networks, and compromise the chemical dopamine and its functionality increases the risk for the onset of Parkinson's disease.

The volume of not only past but also continuing research to determine the cause or causes for Parkinson's disease seems to affirm the statement, quoted above, that Michael J. Fox made to David Letterman in 2015.

"Those you love will go through hard times. Don't give up on them. Patience + Caring + Empathy = Love."

Hallway Poster at the Veterans Administration Outpatient Clinic, Viera, Florida.

7. THOSE AFFECTED

There is a very significant and meaningful community of supporters who are affected after someone receives a confirmed diagnosis for Parkinson's disease. They include the individual's spouse or companion, family members within the home, other family members, neighbors and friends, co-workers, clerics, and supporters within the medical community such as doctors, nurses, clinical staff, therapists and counselors.

Earlier in the narrative, at Chapter 5, "The Diagnosis," there was a description of a rather generalized sequence of events through which someone may obtain a diagnosis for Parkinson's disease. At the onset, the individual himself, immediate members of his family, his neighbors, friends or coworkers may observe physical changes very different from his usual presentation. These changes may be characteristic of some of the symptoms of Parkinson's such as motor impairment.

Normally, an appointment with a doctor follows. A confirmed diagnosis for Parkinson's disease typically is the result of a series of visits, observations and tests by a doctor and a neurologist.

Many spouses frequently accompany their life mates to all of the pre-diagnosis medical appointments. Spouses may be able to help describe and confirm the changes and to elaborate on their characteristics, intensity, frequency and effects. Once at home after having received a confirmed diagnosis, husbands and wives form the primary team to continue their lives together, now with one of the partners living with Parkinson's.

Although Parkinson's is an age-related degenerative disease usually occurring in persons age 60 or older, there may be other persons in addition to the spouse living in the same home. A child, born with a severe disability, who never was able to live alone and care for himself still may live with his elderly parents. One or more senior parents who also cannot live alone and requires help may live within the home. Certainly, persons such as these would be affected.

Extended family members such as siblings, married and single children who no longer live at home, and cousins and grandchildren are among others who are affected. Some of these family members may have skills within the medical community such as doctors, nurses, therapists or care providers and can offer advice or provide personal attention and care.

Some may live close enough to assist maintaining the home and property, and to ease or relieve the primary care provider with his work.

Neighbors and friends are affected in much the same way as extended family members; however, they usually reside much closer and often are in more frequent contact. Their physical location and their ability to support quickly may be the most important factors when the need arises to ask for help.

A person's supporters within the medical community are affected after the confirmed diagnosis through the full progression of the disease. Family doctors, neurologists and their office staffs must remain involved with their patient to deliver the appropriate care. Therapists and counselors often are in closer and more frequent contact with a patient and must establish a rapport to create confidence in the services that they provide and to maintain the patient's motivation to continue with his therapies.

For everyone affected by a person who is living with Parkinson's disease, compassion may be the finest emotion that he can demonstrate. Caring for someone struggling with the debilitating effects of this disease and contributing to that person's vitality and happiness brings out the best of all that is good within us.

The specifics of how this great community

of supporters interact with a person living
with Parkinson's disease are described in the
following two chapters.

"If we do not lay out ourselves in the service of mankind whom should we serve?"

John Adams.   President, The United States of America.

8.   THE MEDICAL COMMUNITY

This morning, Tuesday, July 31, 2018, as I started to write this chapter, I received a telephone call from a very close friend. She was my greatest source of support during the 10 years when I cared for my mother. She called to inform me that she had heard a news broadcast in which Mr. Alan Alda, the multi-talented author, screenwriter and actor, most famous for his role as Doctor Hawkeye Pierce, Captain, United States Army Medical Corps in the television series M*A*S*H, announced that he has received a confirmed diagnosis for Parkinson's disease.

In part, Mr. Alda stated: *"I decided to let people know I have Parkinson's to encourage others to take action. I was diagnosed three and a half years ago, but my life is full. I act. I give talks. If you get a diagnosis, keep moving!"*

Mr. Alda is 82 years old at the time of his announcement. He was just past age 78 when he became symptomatic, was evaluated and received his diagnosis. Born in 1936, the average life expectancy for a white male was just under 60 (59.9), very close to the average age for the onset of Parkinson's disease in males. Having lived for more than 22 years beyond what was guesstimated in the year of his birth as his average life expectancy, Mr. Alda should have every expectation of continued longevity as he lives with Parkinson's.

There is an army of medical professionals who work together with a person living with Parkinson's to help him battle this disease. The purpose of this chapter is to describe the roles of the members of the medical community and how these dedicated professionals serve on behalf of their patients. Those roles include the family medical doctor or health care provider; neurologists; psychiatrists; psychologists; hospital and clinical staff technicians; nurses; physical therapists; speech therapists; dieticians; and, pharmacists.

Medical Doctors.

The family medical doctor or health care provider usually is the first medical professional to evaluate a person who may be symptomatic for Parkinson's. Individuals who are self-employed, others who are employed but may not have health insurance benefits, or those who are retired without health insurance benefits may have a family medical doctor. Individuals who are employed and have health insurance benefits, students, retirees with health insurance benefits and persons who are registered for Medicare and Medicaid may have a health care provider.

As described earlier in Chapter 5, "The Diagnosis," someone who suspects that he may be symptomatic for Parkinson's disease usually will visit his family medical doctor or health care provider first. From the narrative earlier:

"The doctor will listen to his patient's complaints, observe at least one of the early onset symptoms, review his family medical history and conduct a complete medical examination."

He may prescribe medication. If, after all testing and observations, his patient receives a confirmed diagnosis for Parkinson's disease, the doctor may continue to monitor and assess his condition, help plan treatment and therapy, administer medications and provide counseling for diet, exercise and preventative healthcare given the patient's physical condition.

Neurologists.

The second professional, also a medical doctor, who becomes involved with the work to determine a diagnosis, is a neurologist. Again, from the narrative earlier:

"A neurologist is a doctor who is trained to diagnose and treat problems related to the brain and nervous system," and that *"the examination by the neurologist contains all*

of the procedures as those conducted by the family doctor and more."

A neurologist has additional formal medical training; will conduct specific tests with specialized clinical staff; and, will make longer-term observations beyond those of the family medical doctor. Usually it is a neurologist who provides the confirmed diagnosis for Parkinson's disease.

Psychiatrists.

A psychiatrist is a doctor who has completed medical school, a residency, and specializes in mental health. Although most people who have an awareness about Parkinson's because of someone they know who is living with the disease, most people associate Parkinson's with the physical motor symptoms which they are able to observe. However, there are several psychiatric manifestations which are very common and which impair a person's quality of life as severely as his motor symptoms. Some of those psychiatric manifestations include anxiety (affecting between 25 and 45 percent of persons with Parkinson's), depression (affecting as many as 60 percent), delusions, hallucinations, impulse control, paranoia, psychosis and sleep difficulties. Depression, for example, has been described in the research literature as very common in persons with Parkinson's. The research also has demonstrated that there is a pseudo-symbiotic relationship between depression and Parkinson's disease, that is, the presence of one condition increases the risk of the other condition.

As medical doctors, psychiatrists can prescribe anti-anxiety and antidepressant medications. (The potential for possible side effects from these types of medications is described next at Chapter 9, "Management and Control.) Psychiatrists also can conduct psychotherapy, more simply, counseling. This counseling may help someone to understand and overcome negative thoughts and feelings about living with Parkinson's and make attitude and lifestyle changes striving for positive and helpful results.

Psychologists.

A psychologist is a trained professional with the clinical skills to help people identify, understand and cope with issues related to mental health and life status. Although not a medical doctor, a psychologist, similar to a psychiatrist, has studied the brain, its functions and its influence on a person's attitudes, emotions and feelings. However, unlike a psychiatrist, a psychologist cannot prescribe medications.

There is insufficient research to determine which professional provides greater benefit to a person with Parkinson's disease as a result of his counseling. Because of issues such as locations, scheduling appointments, and costs associated with visits to either a psychiatrist or a psychologist, there is evidence that a greater number of persons with Parkinson's who seek counseling will choose a psychologist. Issues such as these, which are related to costs, are described at Chapter 10, "Associated Costs."

Nursing Staff.

Teams of nurses and medical technicians support these doctors. They may work in hospitals, clinics, laboratories, offices, assisted living communities, and nursing care facilities. These nurses and technicians are trained in a variety of skills many of which are overlapping.

Registered Nurses.

Registered Nurses (RN's) are among the most numerous and work with doctors in their offices, hospitals and other medical facilities. Generally, their tasks are related to pre-consult screenings and examinations, patient care, case management and treatment planning. In addition to assisting physicians who provide treatment, they help care for patients. Their duties may include monitoring, recording and reporting symptoms or changes in patient's conditions; maintaining their patients' reports and medical histories; administering medications and treatment, and observing responses, reactions or side effects. Equally important in their support is the health status information which they provide to both the patient and his family.

Nurse Practitioners.

A Nurse Practitioner (NP) is a Registered Nurse who has earned a specialized graduate degree. Most NP's work under the supervision of a doctor as part of a healthcare team or they may work independently. They are trained to order certain diagnostic tests, interpret test results such as those from lab work or x-rays, diagnose diseases, prescribe medications and initiate treatment plans.

Licensed Practical Nurses.

Licensed Practical Nurses (LPN's), like RN's, work in the same types of facilities and support doctors, RN's and NP's. Their tasks usually are less technical, such as taking vital signs, administering injections and providing medications. Many LPN's continue with their formal nursing education to earn degrees as RN's.

Nurse Manager.

Persons may be hospitalized for conditions related to Parkinson's disease before and after they have received a confirmed diagnosis. In the hospital, a patient will receive care from nursing staff supervised by a Nurse Manager. Nurse Managers oversee the nurses on the floor who care for patients. In collaboration with doctors, they perform a variety of duties related directly to patient care and administration including helping the families of their patients.

Staff Nurses.

A Staff Nurse is a RN who is responsible to manage a patient's care. In a hospital or at an outpatient clinic, Staff Nurses care for individuals who are ill or injured. Often, a Staff Nurse is the first healthcare professional to support someone after his arrival at a facility for treatment. In an emergency room, Staff Nurses will hear a person's complaints, assess his condition, obtain vital signs and prepare a summary for a doctor. After care is provided, Staff Nurses support the patient's discharge by providing and explaining post-discharge instructions and supporting the logistics requirements and instructions to the family, if appropriate, at the time of discharge.

Outside of a hospital, in facilities such as a rehabilitation center, assisted living community, nursing home, mental health clinic or critical care center, a Staff Nurse may attend to a person who is living with Parkinson's disease. Like Nurse Managers and other Staff Nurses at a hospital, a Staff Nurse provides direct patient care such as scheduling and coordinating daily tasks, monitoring meals and medications and consulting with doctors and families.

Nurse Case Managers.

A person with Parkinson's disease who is living at home or elsewhere may have the support of a Nurse Case Manager whose role is to evaluate a patient's status and then coordinate a long-term care plan. Usually this work is done from a hospital or a doctor's office. Nurse Case Managers are Registered Nurses who do not perform typical nursing duties but instead serve as coordinators for help for special services such as access to public resources including Medicare and Medicaid, counseling sources, nursing care, health and welfare classes and support groups. This resource is provided primarily for the patient but often includes his family.

Certified Nursing Assistants.

There may be a Home Health Nurse who lives in or visits the home to provide care. This nurse may be supported by a Certified Nursing Assistant (CNA) who helps to provide basic patient care and assist with daily activities. Patient care includes taking vital signs, administering medications and maintaining health records; bathing, dressing and grooming; serving meals, helping a patient to eat or feeding him; and physical support tasks if the patient is immobile or bedridden, such as repositioning (for example, moving or turning while in a bed); transferring (for example, moving between a bed and a wheelchair or between a wheelchair and a toilet); or, transporting (for example, moving between rooms or locations).

This army of medical professionals is reinforced in the battle by additional teams of support professionals. They include physical therapists, speech therapists, dieticians, and pharmacists.

Physical Therapists.

A Physical Therapist is an individual trained in the skills to help persons in need restore and maintain their ideal physical functionality by means of a variety of exercises focused on the limbs and the torso. They typically work in hospitals, private offices and clinics, patients' homes, assisted living facilities and nursing homes. Therapy and exercise routines may be conducted individually by the patient with the observation and supervision of the therapist, or together with assistance from the therapist. The services which are provided are designed and available for anyone in distress from age-related debilitation, illness, accident, injury or surgery with the goal of improving health by restoring functionality and preventing further debilitation.

For persons living with Parkinson's disease, the therapy designed or provided by a Physical Therapist may help to improve balance and range of movement (standing, walking and moving) thereby helping to reduce the risk of falls. Therapies may be designed to include the use of crutches, canes, walkers and wheelchairs in the exercise routines.

Speech Therapists.

A secondary motor symptom which a person living with Parkinson's disease may experience is difficulty with his speech. This arises as a result of the neurodegeneration within the brain which affects the motor control of the muscles in the face and mouth. This compromise or loss of muscle control directly influences and alters speech. This symptom may not affect everyone, and those who are affected may experience different degrees of difficulty.

Speech may be impacted in a variety of ways. They include a softer or gentler tone, a hoarse or raspy quality, a mumbled or slurred expression, a monotone characteristic, or a slowed pace.

A Speech Therapist is a person who is trained to identify, evaluate and treat speech difficulties. His formal training may include education at the Masters level and a year or two of clinical experience. For someone in need, a Speech Therapist will create and implement a personalized treatment plan that addresses his specific functional needs. The therapist is able to assist someone with methods and drills to increase speech volume and rate of speech, focus on annunciation, articulation and clarity, and teach breathing techniques to help amplify and support speech.

Dieticians.

A dietician is a person who is trained to provide nutritional information and advice about what and how to eat in order for a person to achieve or maintain a healthy diet given his physical and medical conditions and life circumstances. A Registered Nutritional Dietician (RND) is a person who has earned a specialized academic degree from an accredited college or university and has served internships or gained work experience from government certified health-care facilities, food-service organizations, military training or internships.

As Parkinson's progresses in a person the muscles in the jaw and mouth become affected, and it becomes more difficult for a person to chew and to swallow food. Information available from a person's doctor, Nurse Case Manager, family members or home health care aides can enable a dietician to create a nutritional plan which describes times for meals and snacks containing a variety of foods and beverages essential and sufficient to meet his nutritional needs and maintain his health.

Pharmacists.

A Pharmacist is a health care professional who is licensed to prepare and dispense drugs and medicines given a written order from a licensed medical practitioner such as a doctor, dentist or advanced practice nurse. In doing so, the Pharmacist must comply with all federal and state drug laws which require him to review and interpret each medical order or prescription, and to detect and prevent any therapeutic incompatibilities with the person's medications.

Pharmacists are an essential resource for persons living with Parkinson's disease. Those persons require a complex regimen of medications to manage symptoms and to provide for functionality. Because no two persons share the same conditions, experience and history with Parkinson's, each person's status is unique. It is for this reason that the skills of a Pharmacist are critical. Knowing a patient, his medical history and his record of medications, the Pharmacist is able to support the medical professionals who prescribe and evaluate the effects of different drugs and their dosages or the combination of different drugs and dosages which are taken simultaneously. Adverse reactions and side effects are another concern for a Pharmacist.

The Pharmacist who knows well a person's medical condition has the ability to provide advice to his doctor for medications when his Parkinson's is compromised by illnesses or infections or by more serious long-term health problems such as dementia or diabetes. Presently, it is medication which is the most effective means by which Parkinson's disease is treated and controlled. For this reason, a person's pharmacist shares a leading role with his doctor in the management of this disease.

One of the miseries suffered by members of the medical community is that on the one hand the professionals know what shocking things can happen to the human body, and on the other hand they also know how very little they can really do about most of them.

The road is long, with many a winding turn,

That leads me to who knows where. . .who knows where.

But I'm strong, strong enough to carry on.

This ain't heavy. It's my passion.

So on I go.

My welfare is my concern.

No burden too great is this to bear.

I'll get there.

For I know that this will not encumber me.

This ain't heavy. It's my passion.

It's a long, long road, from which there is no return.

While I'm on the way to there I will share

That this load will not weigh me down at all.

This ain't heavy. It's my passion.

With sincere apologies to The Hollies for revising a few words of their 1969 hit song, "He Ain't Heavy, He's My Brother."

CHAPTER 9. MANAGEMENT AND CONTROL

I believe that every person who receives a confirmed diagnosis for Parkinson's disease, regardless of his age and status, will resolve to battle the disease with the goal of enjoying the best possible quality of life for the remainder of his life. Over time, I have reinforced that sentiment as a result of the observations I made while caring for my mother for 10 years and working to support other persons living with Parkinson's for 18 years.

The goal of achieving the best possible quality of life is attainable. But it is not easy. It can be accomplished by someone with a positive mental attitude, a passion to achieve his goal and the encouragement and help of his army of supporters.

"This load will not weigh me down at all. This ain't heavy. It's my passion."

People who are passionate about anything in their lives incorporate a daily routine to support that passion. Think athletes with their schedules for practices and play throughout the country; entertainers with their schedules for rehearsals and performances throughout the world; teachers and professors investing hours to prepare lesson plans and more hours dedicated to classroom instruction; astronauts who train for years in the United States, Russia and elsewhere throughout the world to support a space flight mission working in zero gravity while orbiting the earth at 17,500 miles per hour over millions of miles for six months away from their homes and families. This is passion. A disciplined routine is an integral part of any person's passion.

Persons living with Parkinson's disease, who are passionate about attaining and maintaining the best possible quality of life, must develop a new and different lifestyle routine. That routine should include maintaining relationships with family and friends; scheduling regular consultations with doctors who help maintain their health; supporting a regimen for a healthy diet, performing regular physical exercise and therapy; creating a Parkinson's-disease-focused, handicapped-person-friendly physical environment at home; making time for recreation indoors and outdoors; resting (recharging naps and sleep); and, reducing stress. And after all these and other tasks have been planned and conducted there is always one more thing to do.

Most often, a person's family and friends are his greatest sources of support and comfort throughout the battle. Although I cannot quantify this statement from any research on the subject, I suspect that someone living with Parkinson's who has a loving spouse, life-partner or another immediate family member at home with him may have an easier battle to fight than someone who is living alone. Love forms the bond and becomes the driver for an extraordinary level of attention, care and support. For a person living with Parkinson's disease, life will be a constant challenge affecting much of what someone does on a daily basis. The impact of these challenges forces lifestyle changes. A routine or regimen helps to relieve the stress which results from those changes.

A Regimen.

At home, a spouse, partner or family member can provide attention, affection, loving care, and emotional support strengthened by the long-term partnership or family association. These persons are sources for advice, second opinions about courses of action for changes to the lifestyle, and assistance with chores such as commuting, shopping, eating, keeping schedules and appointments, maintaining the home, helping with hygiene, dressing, and supporting exercise, therapy and recreational activities. For everyone living with Parkinson's disease, close personal contacts which come from interacting with someone he loves, helps to provide relief from loneliness, wake up the feel-good chemicals in the brain and contribute to positive, healthy emotions.

After a diagnosis, there now are several reasons to visit with at least three doctors. The first is to continue a relationship with the family doctor and the neurologist to review the general health of the patient and the status of the disease. The second is to support office visits for regular care such as an annual physical and seasonal preventative health care such as immunizations against the flu and pneumonia; and, to consult with the family doctor about any new complaint such as an illness or an injury.

Regular reviews of the status of the disease are very important with both the family doctor and the neurologist. The family doctor will compare records of vital signs to look for any changes that present new threats or problems. He also can review the progress of the symptoms and adjust medications if necessary. Visits for this purpose usually are conducted on a two- or three-month schedule.

The visits with the neurologist may be more involved and lengthier. Ideally, the neurologist will be a doctor who is very experienced working with persons with Parkinson's disease and Parkinsonian-related motor problems. This experience should be the primary reason for selecting him for regular consultations usually on a three- or four-month schedule. He, too, will conduct an examination; evaluate any changes and the progress of existing symptoms; identify new symptoms and their progression; and, determine the effectiveness of the current medications.

Both doctors may make recommendations for additional consultations, tests and therapies. On these occasions, it is very valuable that someone who is living with or has daily or frequent contact with the patient attend the visits. He can help to affirm and supplement the patient's comments and to provide additional new information. At home, he can help incorporate changes or new conditions which were advised by the doctor.

The third doctor is the person's dentist. Regular visits to the dentist, at least twice annually for cleanings, are necessary. A person living with Parkinson's disease needs strong, healthy, well-maintained teeth and good habits for oral hygiene to help sustain his ability to eat and chew solid foods.

Beginning at home, a routine of daily activities performed at certain times (for example, breakfast at 8 a.m.) or for specified times (for example, 30 minutes of therapy each day) helps to make a person living with Parkinson's disease become accustomed to those tasks necessary to achieve the best possible quality of life. The health and status of the person and any conflicts with special occasions may affect the regimen. Windows of opportunity for times in the morning, afternoon or evening may be easier to support than specific times for certain activities.

In Chapter 3, "The Aging Process," I described Mrs. Rath, my 10th grade Biology teacher, explaining genetics and DNA in one class. In another class, I recall her telling us to "Listen to your bodies: sleep when you're tired and get up when you're rested; eat when you're hungry and stop when you're full; do things that give you pleasure and avoid conflict; maximize pleasure and minimize pain; keep company with people who are as good

or better and as smart or smarter than you.".
. .or words to that effect.

Although there may have been difficulties
with sleep during the night, it is important
for someone to wake up feeling somewhat or
fully rested, and leave the bed some time
during the early morning. The early morning
routine of using the facilities and tending
to personal hygiene begins most days. When
possible, the person should change completely
from the clothing worn to bed, and dress
comfortably to start the day.

The act of eating and the chores of chewing
and swallowing may become more difficult as
the disease takes hold of the muscles of the
face and jaws so that breakfast, which begins
the series of daily meals and snacks, should
be simple but complete and easily managed.

Because it is known that no particular food
item or combination of food items has been
proven to help in Parkinson's disease, it is
important to eat a balanced diet, ideally
created with the help of a nutritionist or
dietician. There are, however, certain foods
which may help alleviate the adverse effects
of some of the symptoms. As an example,
consuming foods that are high in fiber and
drinking sufficient fluids, especially water
between breakfast and dinner, can help prevent
constipation, a condition that is common in
persons with in Parkinson's disease.

Medications which are prescribed for "twice
daily" usually are taken the first time during
or after breakfast. Sometime later there may

be the need to return to the bathroom to use the facilities. Then, after washing again, it is important that the person brush his teeth and maintain his daily routine for after-meals oral hygiene. Flossing once in the morning after breakfast and again in the evening after dinner is ideal. At least once a day is essential.

Early mid-morning presents a good time for the first of two daily exercise or physical therapy sessions for between 30 and 45 minutes. The first session for the day should include warm-up stretching and flexibility movements for 10 to 15 minutes followed by light exercise. Stretching and flexibility exercises help with more freedom of movement for regular daily activities such as getting dressed and reaching for objects on a shelf. The exercise routine should engage the brain and stress, but not overload, the body and its muscles used for movement and balance, and strengthen those arm and leg muscles used for gripping, holding, lifting, carrying and moving. In general, exercising may increase a person's muscle strength, flexibility, balance, and can improve overall well-being.

Additional hydration may be needed. Plain water is ideal.

A snack after exercising always is justified. A piece of fruit, a cup of fruit salad, a granola bar or an energy bar with low sugar and low sodium meets the need. General Foods Nature Valley Granola and Protein Bars helped support my mother for more than 10 years and have been my favorite snack for almost 40 years.

Late mid-morning affords time for personal administrative tasks such as responding to mail or telephone messages and organizing for the remainder of the day or week. Depending upon a person's physical status he may continue to perform chores around the home.

There is great value to family and friends having a window during which they know that they may call or otherwise contact their loved one without interrupting his regimen for exercise, meals, hygiene and rest. Once a daily routine is established, a person living with Parkinson's disease should inform his family and friends of the times when he is working through his daily regimen and the times when he is free. This time outside of the regimen, especially outside of meal hours, is the time that he should either initiate or receive calls and messages.

Before the noon meal may be the ideal time for a shower or bath. The time required for this activity also depends upon his physical status with everything from undressing, bathing, dressing and grooming taking longer when someone's assistance is required. But a shower or bath usually is refreshing and relaxing. (On days when exercise or therapy may be planned for a pool then it is not necessary for a late morning shower or bath.)

The noon meal should be full and sufficient and include a protein source, starch, vegetable, and beverage. It is well-justified after an active morning, and provides the energy for the remainder of the day.

Nothing justifies an afternoon nap more than a full and sufficient meal. A rest for 30 to 60 minutes is restorative. A person who may need to nap mid-day longer than 60 minutes may be sleep deprived. This condition should be mentioned to his doctor at his next health check.

If a person is too fatigued given his health status and the stage of the disease then it may not be possible to perform a second session for exercise, therapy or some form of recreation in the afternoon. But if he is motivated and able then, following the nap, early- to mid-afternoon is an ideal time for a second session either indoors or outdoors. The purpose is to continue to engage the brain, stimulate the body, move the torso, and make the muscles work. Movement in a pool is extraordinarily beneficial, working the whole body without much stress.

Active recreation is a productive substitute for physical therapy. Someone living at home would require transportation to places where there are opportunities. Walking along a beach or lakeside, at a park or around a school track breaks up the routine at home. Attending dances or song and dance fests expands someone's circle of friends and works the body in fun ways. Activities with support groups may help someone to learn from others about

102

their experiences and coping techniques, new developments and methods to help manage symptoms, referrals for help, and give a sense of camaraderie among people fighting the same battle.

When I am free from stateside obligations, between the spring and autumn, I like to visit Europe where I maintain a residence. In Italy, especially along the coasts, restaurants usually do not open for dinner before 7 p.m., and customers usually do not arrive before 8 p.m. This is the sort of dinner hour which I really enjoy. However, when I return to the States, I live in Florida (God's Waiting Room) for three to six months of the year. In Florida, the senior citizen community has dinner as early as 4 p.m. and no one who wears a hearing aid, uses a walker or wheelchair, or travels in a vehicle which has been parked in a place designated for the handicapped is still at a restaurant for dinner after 8 p.m.

At a stateside hospital, assisted living facility or nursing home the dinner hours usually are between 4:30 p.m. and 6 p.m.

A person living with Parkinson's usually is a senior citizen who, especially stateside, has his dinner earlier rather than later. After a full day of activity, a senior may have his dinner around 6 p.m. If he has enjoyed a full and sufficient meal at noon, then this meal should be lighter making it easier to digest and not disturb his sleep during the night. Medications which are prescribed for "twice daily" usually are taken for the second time during or after dinner.

103

For persons living with Parkinson's disease, I am an advocate for a small dish of ice cream every evening after dinner. Our taste buds for sweets are the last of the senses which we lose as we age. To me, someone who is battling Parkinson's disease has more health-related issues to be concerned about than his cholesterol numbers. Everyone feels good after eating ice cream.

Persons living with Parkinson's disease deserve to feel good all the time, and ice cream is a great reward at the end of any day – good or bad. I recommend Blue Bell ice cream – any flavor. I am partial to Mint Chocolate Chip; my friend Helen enjoys Cherry Vanilla and Mom's favorite was Homemade Vanilla.

After dinner, it is time to stand down and prepare to end the day. A trip to the bathroom to use the facilities, wash and tend to oral hygiene is necessary. So is a trip to the bedroom to change clothes.

How a person chooses to relax before bedtime should be in a way that makes it easier to bring on restful sleep. Sleep is an important factor to maintain good health. Studies have shown that sleep can help boost the immune system, prevent disease, and ease depression all of which are conditions threatened or exacerbated by the onset of Parkinson's disease. A good night's sleep can be sabotaged by going to sleep at the wrong time, getting too much screen time (television, computer, cell phone) before bed, or self-medicating.

104

But a good night's sleep can be enhanced by praying, meditating, purposefully relaxing, and certainly by shutting down all electronics well before bedtime.

To this end, snacking while watching the television news serves no good. It can generate nightmares in the stomach and in the mind. For someone who enjoys watching television, perhaps an early evening Classic Movie (musicals and comedies are great attention-keepers), a Nature or National Geographic special, or a History Channel documentary may be gratifying. A good book never fails.

Heath Union, which provides support to the website "ParkinsonsDisease.net" described in its newsletter of August 22, 2018, that 72 percent of persons living with Parkinson's (64 of 89 responders) believe that it is "Very Helpful" to follow a daily regimen. That was my experience for ten years.

Attention to the Home.

Anyone who has seen the 2004 movie, *"Million Dollar Baby,"* starring Clint Eastwood and Morgan Freeman, may remember the dialogue between Frankie Dunn, the boxing manager and Maggie Fitzgerald, the prize fighter:

Frankie: *"What's the rule?"*

Maggie: *"Always protect myself."*

Over time, Parkinson's will be responsible for accidents and injuries that further complicate the life of someone living with the

105

disease. Recognizing this threat, it is essential to provide for the protections at home and in the community which will preclude any accident or injury.

Slips and trips are the single greatest cause for injuries especially in the home. Seniors who are living with Parkinson's disease, especially elderly females with osteoporosis and brittle bones, are at an increased risk for injury. Among elderly females it is surprising that frequently it is not known if a woman fell and broke her hip or if her hip broke causing her to fall. Either way, it is a very painful event requiring surgery and long-term physical therapy. An unwillingness or inability to respond to therapy may mean that the person will never walk again.

One of the first actions that should be taken after someone receives a diagnosis for Parkinson's and decides to remain at home to fight the battle is to make a serious review of the physical structure and make changes in the interests of safety.

External lighting should be bright and extend over all of the area that a person will traverse when moving outside the home when it is dark. Automatic light sensors which sense movement and turn on and off automatically are particularly valuable. No one has to search for a light switch, many of which are not easily accessible from a wheelchair or difficult to find in the dark.

Steps are a threat. Outside the home there often are steps from the sidewalk to the walkway leading to the front door and from the alcove at the front door into the home. Occasionally there are steps at other doorways leading into the home. Those steps should be eliminated by the construction of a concrete low-angle incline on which a person can walk and a walker or wheelchair can roll without negotiating steps. If that cannot be done, then posts with grab bars or grab bars alone should be installed to enable someone to negotiate the steps with this type of support.

As Parkinson's strengthens its grip on someone over time, a person will not be able physically to negotiate steps. Inside the home, especially a two-story home, steps are an equal or greater threat to those steps which are outside.

In a two-story home, action should be taken to establish the master bedroom on the ground floor. Overcoming the danger to climbing steps in both directions outweighs the issues of the cost and cosmetic appearance from making a modification. Often there is a step leading into the shower. That step can be overcome by the use of a transfer chair which extends between the outside and inside of the shower.

Grab bars are essential in all bathrooms. There are organizations which will provide free advice and installation of grab bars as a service to senior citizens in need. In a shower, the grab bars should be positioned in a horseshoe shape at various levels and angles. In the bathroom, grab bars should be installed on the wall(s) of one or both sides of the toilet and, if possible, opposite the toilet for gripping when standing. There may be a benefit to a grab bar at either or both sides of the vanity to help with standing from a wheelchair and provide for balance when standing.

Old-fashioned, low-seating toilets make it harder to sit and stand from a sitting position. Taller toilets are more convenient and practical. A portable toilet seat, many of which can be adjusted at the legs to vary the height of the seat, can be used over a fixed low-seating toilet. These seats are built with side arm rests which provide for balance when sitting and help with standing. A portable toilet seat saves the expense of replacing the toilet.

Back to grab bars: elsewhere within the home, a grab bar, different in appearance from those in the bathroom, may have a benefit in the kitchen and the dining room or wherever a person sits for his meals. If eating unassisted, this grab bar can help to provide stability as someone transitions himself to the table and moves a chair to sit.

Over time, a person living at home may require the use of a wheelchair. Most standard doors range in widths from 28 to 32 inches. Medicare-approved manual wheelchairs for someone on the larger side of the height and weight scales are 24 inches. That 24 inches is the width between the left and right wheels of a wheelchair which is somewhat too narrow for many of the bulkier persons who are digging their graves with their teeth. To support these people, many heavy-duty wheelchairs now are wider than 24 inches. Think about the reasons that seats on commuter conveyances such as planes, trains and buses have expanded to accommodate the increasing girth and mass of travelers.

Using a wheelchair to enter a room, especially the bathroom and water closet, should not present an additional challenge to someone living with Parkinson's. Instead, the person, with help from his family if necessary, should make the modifications to the home to accommodate wider doorways long before those doorways are needed.

In the Army, I heard repeatedly and learned for real the statement that, "You win wars by planning to lose them." With respect to wider doorways within the home, consider the problems which could arise if someone should fall and then, after post-hospitalization and rehabilitation, return home and require the use of a wheelchair for an extended length of time or indefinitely. A modification to expand the doorways is worth every penny of the cost. It served me and those persons who helped me care for my mother very conveniently and effectively for 10 years.

Special attention should be given to the bedroom. The bed, regardless of size, with its box spring and fresh, firm mattress, should be the right height from the floor to allow for movement on and off the bed safely and easily. A nearby night table with a good lamp for reading and room to support a telephone, glass of water and incidentals is essential.

Today, everyone except for me owns and uses a Smart Phone. For a person living with Parkinson's disease, I recommend owning first a landline telephone with extensions in at least three locations: the bedroom on the bedside night table, the kitchen and the living room or family room. This is critical when someone must dial 9-1-1 for emergency help. The emergency response system is able to identify the caller's location easily because of the landline and the installation software which supports emergency notification locations. This is not true for a Smart phone or cell phone when someone who, after dialing 9-1-1, must take time to tell the emergency dispatcher his location. Valuable response time is lost when using other than a landline to call 9-1-1.

A person's Smart phone or cell always can be kept with him.

Wall-to-wall carpeting and tile are equally functional for movement throughout the home. Carpet may be warmer and more comfortable to walk on; tile may be easier to move on when using a wheelchair, easier to clean and more appropriate in the bathrooms and kitchen. Throw rugs are a danger and should not be anywhere in the home that is used by a person with Parkinson's. Throw rugs upend and move too easily. They present a serious risk for slipping and tripping.

Clothing and footwear should be functional, comfortable and easy to put on, adjust and remove. Looser clothing is easier for dressing because there is little or no tension when fastening buttons or using zippers. Large buttons are preferable to smaller ones for ease of use with fingers and hands that may have lost their flexibility.

Shoes and sneakers which can be fastened with Velcro are easier for a person to use when dressing himself. So is footwear such as moccasins or Docker-style loafers which simply slip on for wearing.

Socks, briefs and undershirts should be loose-fitting and easy to put on and remove.

T-shirts, daily wear business casual shirts (short- or long-sleeved shirts with a collar), and dress shirts should be cotton or other material which can be washed easily by machine. Shorts and trousers should be cotton, wool or polyurethane that also are easily washable by machine. Some dress slacks should be dry cleaned. It is helpful to check the clothing labels for washing instructions.

A person's vital signs, blood work and health status are the best indicators for what foods and beverages a person consumes. An estimated 160 million Americans (about half the population of the United States) are either obese or overweight. Nearly 75 percent of American men and more than 60 percent of

American women are obese or overweight. Within that group, the greatest prevalence of obesity and overweight was found among men aged 50 to 54 (80 percent) and women aged 60 to 64 (73 percent), ages which are closing in on the average age for the onset of Parkinson's disease.

Troubles with most people seem to come by the pound. Imagine being obese and living with Parkinson's disease. How do you get in and out of bed? How do you get on and off the toilet? How difficult is it for you to tend to your personal hygiene when showering or bathing? How do you keep all of your mass clean and germ free? How do you move? Do you need a wheelchair? If so, what size? How are you transported? How do you exercise to improve your mobility? How much longer does it take you to accomplish basic chores? How many persons does it take to help you do things that you could be doing for yourself if you were not obese? Are you inviting or do you already have diabetes which complicates all other health issues besides Parkinson's disease? Where is your sense of self-respect? Do you want to die young, maybe younger than your parents or grandparents? Do you think that being obese is how we as humans were meant to evolve?

It is inappropriate and incorrect to write that there is an ideal diet, and similarly to suggest that one diet fits all. However, with respect to diet, there are two caveats which ring true: "Don't eat anything that comes out of a box or a bag," and, "If it tastes good, spit it out."

Now, it is important to stress than anyone who is living with Parkinson's disease and who is overweight or obese seek counseling from a certified dietician or nutritionist, and do everything physically possible, shy of surgery, to lose the excess weight. Being overweight or obese compromises your ability to take the actions necessary to battle this disease. Living with Parkinson's disease may be enough suffering for one person. No one should not have to suffer needlessly from the adverse effects on the body as a result of being overweight or obese.

"Living with a terminal illness is a process."

Mrs. Ronald Garan. Former United States Air Force nurse. Clear Lake, Texas neighbor and friend.

10. ONSET TO DEATH.

Every human being is capable of loving, learning, teaching, growing and inspiring until the very end of his life. A person living with Parkinson's disease is no exception. Michael J. Fox, husband, father and former child-star entertainer, who received a diagnosis for early-onset Parkinson's disease in 1991 at age 29, has been doing all of this on his own and through the Michael J. Fox Foundation for Parkinson's Research. Michael announced his diagnosis and status in 1998, two years before I began to care for my mother. She was my source for loving and growing; Michael and his foundation are my sources for learning, and being inspired.

I am not able to generalize at what time and

114

with what sentiment a person who has received a diagnosis for Parkinson's disease makes his decision about how to accept the diagnosis and how to move forward. From research-related interviews, many persons have stated that their first concerns were not for themselves but for their spouses and their families and what will happen to them.

Independence at the early stages.

Unless issues of memory loss or dementia accompany someone's diagnosis, persons who are living with Parkinson's disease may be able to care for themselves and manage their affairs for months or years with only occasional or part-time help. Few people, for any reason, willingly or easily give up their freedom or their independence. (I think this may be the reason that there are vows at most marriage ceremonies.) Having received a diagnosis for Parkinson's, most people, regardless if they are living alone or with someone else or others, prefer to continue to do as much as possible for as long as possible for themselves before they seek assistance.

When someone first becomes symptomatic, for example, with motor issues such as tremor, balance problems or difficulty walking, he usually assumes a physical or situational irregularity which will go away. The younger a person is, the more likely that this is true. The symptoms which appear at the early onset of the disease usually are not severe, and rarely do not occur regularly or with the same intensity.

It is only when a tremor does not go away, when it repeats itself more frequently and more severely, and when someone else alerts him to the condition about which he already knows, that a person takes the first step to consult a doctor.

The initial visit to a doctor and additional visits to other doctors and specialists may conform to the diagnostic routine described earlier in the five pages of Chapter 5, "The Diagnosis." Often this is a lengthy process, extending over several weeks or months, before a diagnosis for Parkinson's disease is confirmed. This diagnostic process provides the time for someone symptomatic to assume the worst and to begin planning accordingly. Probably not act, but certainly plan. The winds of war are blowing and, consistent with the military maxim that, "You win wars by planning to lose them," there is great value for someone who suspects that he may be symptomatic to assemble those most devoted to him and begin planning for battle in a war that cannot be won.

After receiving a confirmed diagnosis, it is time to act on the plan. What everyone who has received this diagnosis should know and understand at that time, if not before, is that Parkinson's is a progressive degenerative disease; that the symptoms will become worse, not better; and, that during his lifetime he will be completely dependent upon others to support him at the latest stages of the disease.

During the early stages, a person newly-diagnosed with Parkinson's often is able to care for himself and maintain his lifestyle. The symptoms and their degree of severity tend to determine his status. It seems to be true that a person in high spirits feels better and heals quicker than another.

If employed, he may continue to work. There may be issues or threats if he drives to work or anywhere else. What is the commuting distance and how congested is the traffic during the commute? Medications may cause drowsiness; his reaction time to unexpected events may have slowed; he may have spasms or spontaneous contractions which make it difficult to grasp a steering wheel, work turn signals or windshield wipers; move his foot quickly between the gas pedal and the brake, or keep his foot firmly on the brake and stay stopped. If his eye muscles are weakened then his peripheral vision and depth perception may be compromised and present a threat to driving. Having described this, only the person himself with input from others can evaluate the merits of his ability to drive safely. If his ability to drive a vehicle has been compromised by the disease then so, too, may be his capability to deliver productive work. If so, then this as an issue, is moot.

If not employed, then there is far less activity for someone to accomplish on his own during the day. A generalized list and description of those activities are described in Chapter 9, "Management and Control," at the first section, "A Regimen."

After diagnosis and for the first five to seven years of the initial three stages, a person living with Parkinson's disease still is relatively physically independent.

Dependence at the middle stages.

As Parkinson's progresses through the middle stages, the severity of symptoms increases from mild to moderate. When the symptoms worsen as the disease seizes greater control of a person's body, the need arises for help with routine daily tasks which have become too difficult or too time-consuming.

It may be as difficult for someone in need to ask for help outside of his family as it is for someone to provide it. Caregiving is always difficult. Daily living can present more than sufficient sources of stress. Add to that the responsibility of caring for a spouse, parent, sibling or other family member or close friend who needs care and the stress of being a caregiver can be overwhelming. In this mid-stage, as the need for care for an increasing number of tasks becomes a reality, there is a heightened awareness among everyone involved that Parkinson's truly is a degenerative disease. The person himself may have this awareness, and how he responds physically and emotionally affects those who help provide his care.

One of the early needs to satisfy is to secure reliable transportation when someone is unwilling or unable to drive safely. There

118

are at least two reasons to do this. The first is that a substitute driver could protect his safety and the safety of the public. The second is that a substitute driver could provide for his access to doctors, therapists, family, friends, grocery shopping, or provide a change of environment for exercise or recreation all of which may require a commute.

Most persons living with Parkinson's disease and those people closest to them usually have observed significant improvement in the control of symptoms after beginning treatment with medications. But over time, however, the benefits of those medications frequently diminish or become less consistent. As the disease progresses the classic symptoms may increase in number, in intensity or both. When this happens, the medications which are used to control symptoms may have to be modified either by altering their dosages, increasing their frequency, or adding new medications.

Any changes may cause side effects which adversely affect the physical abilities and emotional stability of the person. Bouts of depression can lead to withdrawal from essential activities that support the battle such as eating and exercising regularly.

Within the senior citizen community a certain melancholy and a certain irascibility may characterize the aging process. Many families sense that ill-temper accompanies advancing age. When a person begins to break down emotionally then everyone who is associated with his care is affected.

Disrespectful conduct and demonstrations of frustration such as rage tend to discourage anyone's willingness to help, especially if the help is provided as a favor. When a paid caregiver quits providing a service, the person or his family must find a qualified and acceptable replacement. This is a difficult and often time-consuming task.

As Parkinson's progresses through the middle stages a person living with the disease at home will require more help with more of his daily tasks. But during these middle stages, the degree of disability and the need for assistance does not rise to that for someone totally disabled, bedridden and requiring attention and care around the clock.

Total dependence at the final stages.

During the final stages, the severity of the symptoms increases from moderate to severe.

Beyond the need for a driver at the early and middle stages, and perhaps with the same level and frequency of support, there now will be a need for assistance with using a walker or wheelchair; help with personal hygiene and bathing; preparing and eating meals; performing exercise and therapy routines that improve flexibility and maintain strength; managing personal and family financial affairs; housekeeping; and, maintaining the physical property at the residence.

This year, within the United States, there are approximately 40 million unpaid care providers. They include spouses, former spouses (somewhat rare), domestic partners, other family members such as siblings, adult children and grandchildren. Outside of the family, unpaid care providers include neighbors, friends, coworkers, support group volunteers, and church and civic group members. Approximately 60 percent of caregivers are women in their mid-forties and approximately 30 percent of family caregivers are seniors caring for other seniors who are 65 or older.

Paid care providers may be recruited by recommendations from doctors, community local Parkinson's disease support groups, other persons living with Parkinson's, insurance providers, employment websites, and elsewhere. Different needs for help require different skills and abilities. Accordingly, the rates for compensation will vary consistent with extra pay for extra responsibility.

For all the conditions which require physical assistance at home or in a care facility, such as help with movement, hygiene, dressing, shopping, cooking, eating, exercising and socializing, it is important that family and friends closest in relationship to the person receiving the care are aware of his level of comfort and satisfaction with the help or service which is provided.

In the final stages of life for a person living with Parkinson's disease there are quality-of-life care issues which are provided by others. They merit monitoring by his family or friends and feedback from the person himself as well as his care providers. Feedback is helpful for issues such as patient and caregiver attitudes and amicability; personal satisfaction and appreciation for the care; appearance and functionality of everything within the home environment; and, personal safety and physical security. There must be an exceptional degree of trust and confidence with anyone in any capacity who provides unobserved and unsupervised care and support for someone unable to care for himself and completely dependent upon others for a happy, healthy and dignified life while living with Parkinson's disease.

Life can sustain itself long after a person is no longer able to walk, no longer able to communicate, no longer able to care for himself. At this late stage, perhaps as early as seven to 10 years or as late as 20 years or more after diagnosis, the body begins to shut down. There is no longer an interest, willingness or ability to consume foods in any form. After eating stops, the same becomes true for consuming liquids. Natural death is approaching and family members and close friends should be near their loved one.

The death certificate will not describe "Parkinson's disease" as the "Cause of Death." That is because Parkinson's is not a killer disease. Instead, the cause may be described as "malnutrition," or "dehydration," or a dementia-related disease such as Alzheimer's which may accompany Parkinson's and is a killer disease.

English poet John Donne wrote:

"Any man's death diminishes me,

Because I am involved in mankind.

And therefore, never send to know for whom the bell tolls;

It tolls for thee."

"No disease suffered by a man can be known, for every living person has his own peculiarities and always has his own peculiar, personal, novel, complicated disease, unknown to medicine -- not a disease of the lungs, liver, skin, heart, nerves, but a disease consisting of one of the innumerable combinations of the maladies of those organs."

Count Leo Tolstoy, Russian author of War and Peace (1869) and Anna Karenina (1877).

11. ASSOCIATED COSTS.

The statement by Lyov Tolstoy more than 100 years ago remains relevant today to this narrative about Parkinson's disease. Because Parkinson's is primarily an age-related degenerative disease with the average age of onset at 60, persons who receive a diagnosis already may be challenged by other physical and medical complications. In the United States approximately 75 percent of men and more than 60 percent of women are obese or overweight. Obesity has been linked to such serious medical conditions as cancer, diabetes, gallbladder disease, gout, heart disease, high blood pressure, osteoarthritis, and stroke. Accordingly, there is a 50 percent or greater chance that a person, age 60 or older, who receives a diagnosis for Parkinson's disease, also may be overweight or obese and, if so, suffering from one or more of these obesity-related conditions. For this reason, it is very difficult to calculate the costs associated with living with Parkinson's disease.

The progressive disability associated with Parkinson's combined with the possibility, if not the probability, of other medical conditions, result in substantial financial burdens for persons living with the disease and often for their families. On April 19, 2018, Fidelity Investments estimated that a 65-year-old couple who retired that year needed $280,000 to fund their future medical costs above those costs covered by their Medicare premiums. That amount does not include any cost for long-term care. It does include the costs for deductibles, copayments and insurance premiums for coverage for doctor visits, out-of-pocket expenses for prescription drugs, and expenses not covered by Medicare such as hearing aids and eyeglasses. A majority of seniors need and use eyeglasses especially for reading. Many seniors need hearing aids but use them only if they can afford to buy them. The $280,000 figure increased from the 2017 estimate of $275,000, representing a two percent increase. Health care may be one of the largest expenses in someone's retirement budget. A study by HealthView Services determined that the average monthly health care expense for a couple at age 65 is $583. By the age of 85, that number may more than double to over $1,160.

The statistics.

The website, www.payingforseniorcare.com, generated a number of interesting and surprising statistics on the subject of "Long Term Care in the United States" from several sources including the following: AARP Beyond 50; The American Association of Geriatric Psychiatry; The American Association for Long-Term Care Insurance; The Centers for Disease Control and Prevention; The MetLife Market Survey of Nursing Home and Home Care Costs; Standard and Poor's; The United States Congressional Budget Office; The United States Department of Health and Human Services; and, The United States Census Bureau. Those statistics revealed that:

- The chance that an American today is over 65 is one in eight.
- The chance that an American over 65 has no natural teeth is one in four.
- The percentage of all federal domestic spending that goes to the elderly is 46 percent.
- The average annual health care costs for older Americans who earn more than $30,000 a year is $11,000.

- The average annual health care costs for older Americans earning less than $10,000 a year is $17,000.
- The ratio of women over 65 to men over 65 is 1.37 to 1.00.
- The ratio of women over 85 to men over 85 is 2.1 to 1.00.
- The chance that a senior citizen will become physically or cognitively impaired in his lifetime is two in three.
- The chance that a senior citizen will enter a nursing home is one in three.
- The chance that a patient in a nursing home in the United States is sedated or physically restrained is one in two.
- The average cost to stay in a nursing home in the United States for one year is $76,680.
- The average number of days which individuals who require long term care actually receive it are 904.
- The percentage of the older population who has long term care needs and who live at or near the poverty level is 40 percent.
- The percentage of total long-term care hours that are provided by unpaid caregivers is 84 percent.
- The percentage of Americans over 60 who live with a younger relative is 6.3 percent.
- The percentage increase by 2040 in the number of elderly persons who will require long term care and who have no

children to help provide for that care is 50 percent.

- The average number of drugs prescribed each year to an American over age 60 is 16.
- The chance that a senior citizen in the United States reports having skipped his medications or having not filled his prescriptions because of the cost is one in five.
- The chance that an individual will have more than $25,000 in out-of-pocket long-term care costs is one in five.
- The chance that an individual age 55 or older has long-term care insurance is one in 10.
- The percentage of men over age 65 who are married and whose spouse still is living is 73 percent.
- The percentage of women over age 65 who are married and whose spouse still is living is 42 percent.
- The median income for men over age 65 is $24,000.
- The median income for women over age 65 is $14,000. Because women live longer, a 65-year-old woman can expect to spend $22,000 more in total health care costs over the course of her retirement than a man her same age.
- The estimate of total expenditures from the age of 65 until death increase substantially with longevity. That

estimate averages from $40,000 for persons who die at the age of 65 to more than $240,000 for those who die at the age of 90, due, in part, to the high costs of nursing home care.

- The chance that a woman in the United States who is age 75 or older lives alone is one in two.
- The percentage of unpaid or informal caregivers who are women is 75 percent.
- The increase in the average life expectancy of a person in the United State between 1900 and 2000 was 30 years.
- The percentage of leisure time that persons in the United States who are age 65 or older spend watching TV is 55 percent.
- The percentage of leisure time that persons in the United States who are age 65 or older spend exercising is only three percent.

OUCH!

Medicare and Medicaid.

In July 2016, WXEL PBS in South Florida broadcast that, for the first time, the average cost of Medicare per person in the United States exceeded $10,000 annually. The report stated that a stronger economy, faster growth in medical prices and an aging population were responsible for the continuing increased costs. Also, only about five percent of the population who are the most frail, ill or disabled accounts for nearly half the Medicare spending in any given year.

Medicare does help for individuals with Parkinson's disease. Because there is no singular, conclusive medical test to confirm a diagnosis for Parkinson's, the diagnostic process can be lengthy, often requiring multiple visits to more than one doctor. These visits are covered by Medicare at only 80 percent of the approved cost until the person's deductible is met.

Outside the Medicare-provided medical assistance, in the non-medical areas, Medicare provides almost no help. It does not pay for personal care at home, in assisted living or in adult day care facilities. Medicare also does not provide for assistance with the activities of daily living except when those activities are provided in a nursing home. Medicare's nursing home benefit is limited to partial coverage for a maximum of 100 days which is absolutely insufficient once the need for that type of care has been validated. Medicare does offer a home care benefit but only for at-home health care and not for at-home personal care.

Original Medicare consists of two parts: Part A and Part B. The following information is relevant only if medical services or supplies are obtained from a Medicare-authorized provider after certification from the doctor.

There is no premium for Medicare Part A (Hospital insurance) if a person has worked and paid Medicare taxes for at least 10 years or 40 quarters. In 2018, someone who did not qualify for premium-free Medicare Part A may have had to pay as much as $400 a month. Then, someone who may require an inpatient hospital stay would pay a Medicare Part A deductible of $1,340 for each benefit period, plus coinsurance depending upon the length of the hospitalization. "Coinsurance" is a percentage of a health care service for which a person is responsible. During the first 60 days of a hospitalization, there is no coinsurance cost. Then, between day 61 to day 90 the coinsurance cost is $335 per day. From day 91 and beyond the coinsurance cost jumps to $670 for each "lifetime reserve day" for each benefit period. A Medicare recipient is entitled to only 60 "lifetime reserve days" after which he becomes responsible for all hospitalization costs.

There are additional costs associated with care in a skilled nursing facility. Similar to hospitalization costs, there is zero coinsurance cost for the first 20 days of each benefit period. That cost jumps to $167.40 per day between days 21 and 100. After day 100, a Medicare recipient is responsible for all costs.

Medicare Part B is medical insurance for which there is a monthly premium which is deducted from someone's Social Security benefits. A Medicare recipient eligible for Part B before 2018 pays an average of $130 – $135 for this premium. Many retirees may opt to purchase Medigap policies which provide coverage in addition to what is offered through Medicare or Medicare Part D (Prescription drug coverage).

To keep costs down for the facility and the patient, many doctors, hospital and skilled nursing care facility managers try to limit patient stays to the shortest number of days in the first benefit period when there is no coinsurance cost. A more detailed description of these and other costs as well as other services provided through Medicare can be found online at the website: www.medicare.gov.

Private Insurance.

In the text from eHealth's Health Insurance Price Index Report for 2016, was the statement that individuals between the ages of 55 and 64 who purchased private insurance without a government subsidy paid an average of $580 a month for premiums. In that same report, premiums for individual coverage averaged $321 per month. Premiums for family plans averaged $833 per month. The average annual deductible for individual plans was $4,358 and the average annual deductible for family plans was $7,983. Persons living with Parkinson's disease will not have all of their disability-related medical costs paid for by Medicare. There may be a need for supplemental health insurance which should be determined by the person and his family immediately after receiving the diagnosis for Parkinson's.

Doctors and Dentists.

In Chapter 9, "Management and Control" the

narrative described the need and provided some justification for a person living with Parkinson's disease to maintain regular contact with his doctors and dentist. For persons age 65 or older with Medicare many of the expenses associated with a visit to a doctor are paid for by Medicare. But Medicare does not cover most dental care, procedures, or supplies. Cleanings, fillings, extractions crowns, bridges, dentures, dental plates, or other dental devices are not covered. The exception is that Medicare Part A (Hospital Insurance) does pay for certain dental services provided when someone is hospitalized. A person living with Parkinson's who is younger than 65 must rely on private insurance to help defray the cost of visits to a doctor. In this case, there are costs usually not covered by private insurance such as deductibles and co-payments for which the individual is responsible.

Transportation.

When a person living with Parkinson's disease has determined either on his own or together with the advice of his closest family members or friends that he is no longer able to drive safely then there may be costs associated with his transportation to provide for services such as driving to medical appointments and therapy sessions, and to satisfy needs or interests such as banking, grocery shopping or recreation away from the home. Often a family member or friend will help. But without someone then there is the cost for safe and reliable transportation.

These costs vary because of a number of driver compensation factors such as the day and time, round-trip distance, fuel expenditure, waiting time, and associated labor if any. Many senior citizen, veterans and support group organizations have volunteers who may be available to provide service without charge.

Medications, Vitamins and Supplements.

Persons living with Parkinson's disease may require a variety of different medications and at different dosages to manage their symptoms. These medications serve to manage symptoms by substituting for or increasing the production of dopamine in the brain. But, over time these medications may become less effective requiring either increased dosages, new medications or both. Additional medications present the problem of additional costs.

Medicare Parts A and B may not cover prescription medications. Normally, Medicare Part A covers only medications provided when someone is an inpatient in a hospital or other facility. Medicare Part B may cover medications which are administered inside a clinic. Typically, Medicare Parts A and B do not cover medications which are taken at home. In this case, the person would need coverage through Medicare Part D (Prescription Drug Plan) private retirement insurance to pay for these medications. The premiums for Medicare Part D and supplemental insurance are determined by the providers. They will differ not only by plan but also by the geographical area in which the insured resides. Premiums for Medicare Part D and supplemental insurance are expensive and would add significantly to anyone's health care budget.

With respect to private insurance, most insurance plans pay a portion of the medications only after someone has met his deductible. This requirement results in expensive out-of-pocket costs which vary by the number, types and dosages of the medications.

In addition to medications, vitamins and supplements which support a healthful diet may help with the management and control of the disease. Studies have validated the benefit to reducing toxic load and homocysteine. Homocysteine is an amino acid which, when elevated in the body, becomes toxic. It has been shown to be elevated in people living with Parkinson's disease. Homocysteine levels can be reduced with folic acid, vitamins B12 and B6, zinc and tri-methyl-glycine (TMG). Some of these nutrients are co-factors for dopamine production. Magnesium is a mineral that acts as a natural relaxant and may help with Parkinson's-related issues such as constipation, high blood pressure, insomnia, irregular heartbeat, muscle tremors or spasms, and sleep disturbances. Omega-3 fatty acids, which are found in fish such as anchovies, herring, mackerel, salmon, sardine and trout, are anti-inflammatory and mood-boosting nutrients.

Many people living with Parkinson's have a

history of taking dietary supplements before the onset of the disease to help with their nutrition and overall health. However, to date, there are no dietary supplements which have been proven to slow the progression of Parkinson's disease. Some supplements may interfere with medications and should not be taken. In all cases, beyond those medications prescribed by his doctor, a person living with Parkinson's should consult his doctor, pharmacist and nutritionist before adding any vitamins and supplements to his diet.

Physical Therapists.

In Chapter 8, "The Medical Community," there is the statement that Physical Therapists provide services "which are designed and available for anyone in distress from age-related debilitation, illness, accident, injury or surgery with the goal of improving health by restoring functionality and preventing further debilitation," and that "for persons living with Parkinson's disease, the therapy designed or provided by a Physical Therapist may help to improve balance and range of movement (standing, walking and moving) thereby helping to reduce the risk of falls. Therapies may be designed to include the use of crutches, canes, walkers and wheelchairs in the exercise routines."

Physical Therapists are expensive. The average salary for a physical therapist in the United States is $86,520 a year which equates to $7,210 per month, $1,663 per week and

$41.59 per hour. After a hospitalization for an accident or injury, there may be rehabilitation provided by a Physical Therapist and paid for by Medicare in a clinic, facility or at a person's home.

A person living with Parkinson's may decide that physical therapy is necessary for his well-being and employ someone privately. When this happens, it is helpful for a family member or friend to observe, or even to videotape, the therapy. Then, therapy sessions can be conducted in the future using the techniques demonstrated by the trained professional Physical Therapist but conducted by or with the assistance of a family member or friend without cost.

Home Health Care Aides.

Home Health Care Aides are to a person at home much in the way that Certified Nursing Assistants are to patients in a hospital or facility. They provide basic care and administer to a person's needs to do or help him do what he cannot do for himself. But Home Health Care Aides are paid significantly less than Certified Nursing Assistants. The average salary for a Home Health care Aide is between $16,500 and $29,500 per year. On an hourly wage, those salaries equate to only $7.89 and $14.15 per hour respectively.

This is so wrong! How can any adult support a system where his child can earn $15 an hour to flip a burger or make a milkshake yet someone who bathes, clothes, feeds and monitors his sibling, parent or grandparent can command only half that amount? The reason is that these costs which should be paid for by Medicare, Medicaid and other resources within the government are not funded. The final Chapter 14, "Rise Up!" is a call to action on health care issues such as this.

Private Memberships: Gyms and Pools.

Both gyms and pools provide outstanding opportunities to manage and control the physical debilitations associated with living with Parkinson's. Memberships are relatively inexpensive, between $30 and $50 a month, given the opportunity for daily exercise and the benefits gained from such exercise. Among the least expensive gyms, LA Fitness and most local YMCA's have pools suitable for water aerobics, water-resistance exercise and lap swimming. In addition to costs for a membership, there could be additional related expenses such as a driver for transportation and a person to assist with mobility, exercise support and dressing.

Recreation.

There are dozens of activities, many of which are free, by which a person living with Parkinson's disease can participate for the benefit of improving his physical condition and state of mind. Activities which someone finds invigorating helps generate health-enhancing endorphins which help reduce symptoms of depression.

Most doctors know that the mind can do

astonishing things to the body, including suggest false pregnancies. The effect of the mind on the body is extraordinarily great. Good spirits help to recover the lost energies of the body. Consider the brain as a muscle. Like the muscles of our bodies, it is essential to exercise the brain or it will atrophy.

This is especially important for someone who is homebound but who has a family member, friend or group support volunteer who is able to support an activity that exercises the body or stimulates the mind (or both) outside of the home. The first consideration is to identify an activity with which a person has an interest. The second consideration is to fit that activity with the person's health status ensuring that he has the ability and energy to participate.

Some activities which are relatively easy to support are mid-day meals outdoors in a picnic-style environment. Snacking and people-watching at a beach, lake or park breaks up the monotony at home. Watching a college or high school sporting event is exciting, and the chaos which reigns during a children's T-ball baseball game always is fun in the image of a Keystone Cops comedy. Local Performing Arts Centers, community civic, veterans and group support organizations sponsor concerts, music festivals, dances, arts and crafts displays, seasonal and holiday parties which are inexpensive forms of entertainment. Local libraries host authors who describe their personal experiences related to a book which they have written. Others lecture about self-help issues on a variety of subjects, places of interest for travel, or subjects which the library directors determined may have an interest for their patrons and the community.

Home Modifications.

The narrative within Chapter 9, "Management and Control," describes the need and justification for making modifications to the home to provide for the safety, comfort, convenience and functional abilities of someone living with Parkinson's. The costs for some of these modifications can be expensive: building concrete wheelchair ramps which lead into the home; expanding the widths of doorways to permit movement with a wheelchair; installing motion-sensor lighting. Others, such as installing grab bars in the bathroom, showers and tubs, are much less expensive. But every modification necessary to support the at-home residence of someone living with Parkinson's is worth the expense to provide for the happiness of someone who wants to live at home.

"There should be no boundaries to human endeavor. We are all different. However bad life may seem, there is always something you can do and succeed. While there's life, there is hope."

Stephen Hawking, (1942 - 2018), Theoretical physicist and author.

12. NOTABLE AND QUOTABLE.

This chapter provides a narrative about six persons, three men and three women, all of whom enjoy international reputations as persons of accomplishment and all of whom have received a diagnosis for Parkinson's disease. The men are champion boxer and activist Muhammed Ali; actor, author and activist Michael J. Fox; and, Pope John Paul II. The women are actress Deborah J. Kerr; Attorney General Janet Reno; and, photographer and photojournalist Margaret Bourke-White. Among the men, Muhammad Ali and Pope John II are deceased. All three women are deceased.

For all six persons, there is a description of their childhood and early life, their career or profession up to the time of the diagnosis; and, the interests and activities following the diagnosis.

There were numerous notable men from within a variety of professions such as actors, athletes, authors, businessmen, clergy, doctors, entrepreneurs, military leaders and politicians. There were not as many notable women in as many career fields as the men perhaps because it is only recently that women have made deep advances into careers different from entertainers, singers and songwriters. Rather fortunate for the newer female titans of business and industry, I know of none who has received a diagnosis for Parkinson's disease.

Muhammed Ali. (1942 – 2016)

"Impossible is just a word thrown around by men who find it easier to live in the world they've been given than to explore the power they have to change it. Impossible is not a fact. It's an opinion." MA

Muhammad Ali was born Cassius Clay on January 17, 1942 in Louisville, Kentucky to parents Cassius Clay, Sr., a painter and artist and Odessa Clay, a mother, homemaker and occasional part-time laborer as a cook and housekeeper. His brother, Rudolph, was born in 1944.

In this part of the country, society still

was segregated between whites and blacks according to the Old South traditions of Jim Crow. This is especially shameful given the fact that the United States entered World War II in December 1941, only one month before his birth, following the despicable attack by the Japanese at Pearl Harbor. Hundreds of black sailors, Marines, soldiers and airmen perished. After the attack, thousands more blacks enlisted or were drafted and served during the war with distinction. Thousands were wounded or killed. Hundreds of blacks returned wearing Purple Hearts and decorations for valor.

In school, Cassius Clay was an accomplished athlete although he was not distinguished academically. In high school he graduated 376th in a class of 391. He took up boxing as his sport because he knew that to play football or basketball nationally he probably would need the recognition earned from college play. He also knew that a boxer needed only access to a gym, motivation, desire, aptitude and endurance to succeed.

He fought his first match as a young, 13-year old teenager. He and his opponent each weighed only 89 pounds. Clay won in a split decision.

His early training routine had him waking before five in the morning to run several miles, then spend most of the remainder of the day at the gym to workout, train and spar. He developed a professional's training routine while still only a teenager. Exceptionally self-confident, over time he proved himself to be skilled as a boxer, demonstrating strength, speed, agility and skills that he described made him "float like a butterfly and sting like a bee."

His amateur boxing record at age 18 was 100 wins and only eight losses as well as two national Golden Gloves championships. At the same age in the 1960 Summer Olympics in Rome, he won the gold medal for boxing in the finals after a unanimous decision against his Polish opponent. He returned to the United States and turned professional. Over 21 years, he won 56 fights and lost five. He remains the only three-time world heavyweight champion.

In the chaos of the 60's, Cassius Clay became a Muslim and changed his name to Muhammad Ali in what he considered was a demonstration of support for the oppressed minorities. In the mid-60's he refused to be drafted into the military claiming religious objections and opposition to the war in Vietnam. That action resulted in his arrest, conviction of draft evasion and loss of his boxing titles. The conviction was overturned five years later in 1971.

In 1984, three years after retiring from boxing at age 39, Muhammad Ali was diagnosed with Parkinson's disease. In Chapter 6, "Possible Causes," there is the statement that "several studies have concluded that head trauma is a risk factor for neurodegenerative disorders." Although both Muhammad Ali and his personal physician stated that the head trauma which he received after more than 25 years as a boxer was not the cause; certainly, after another 30 years of investigations and studies, there is sufficient evidence to suggest that the head trauma may have been one trigger for the onset of the disease.

Later, in the 1990's, Muhammad Ali became a serious advocate for research about Parkinson's disease. His annual Celebrity Fight Night raised an estimated $100 million for research, a good portion of which was provided by donations from Muhammad Ali himself. In 1997, he and his supporters established the "Muhammad Ali Parkinson Center" located at the Barrow Neurological Institute" which is dedicated to research about Parkinson's disease. As a result of this research, many Research and Care centers, including the Muhammad Ali Parkinson Center, now integrate physical and mental exercise into the treatment of patients.

Thirty-six years after clinching an Olympic gold medal in Rome in 1960, Muhammad Ali's trembling hand lit the 1996 Summer Olympic Flame during the opening ceremony in Atlanta, Georgia. Three years later in 1999, Sports Illustrated named him the "Sportsman of the Century" at its 20th Century Sports Awards ceremony in Madison Square Garden in New York City.

Describing him the greatest boxer of all time, President George W. Bush presented him the Medal of Freedom in a ceremony at the White House in 2005.

In the final stages of the disease, Muhammad Ali was cared for by his family and died with them in Scottsdale, Arizona on June 3, 2016. The cause of death was septic shock. He was 74 years old.

"If my mind can conceive it and my heart can believe it then I can achieve it." MA

Michael J. Fox.

"We may each have our own individual Parkinson's, but we all share one thing in common. Hope." MJF

Michael Andrew Fox was born on June 9, 1961 in Edmonton, Alberta, Canada to parents William Fox, a law enforcement officer and member of the Canadian Armed Forces and Phyllis Piper Fox, an actress and finance clerk. He is the fourth of five children in his family which includes a brother and three sisters. He and his family relocated within Canada while his father was assigned with the Armed Forces finally settling in Burnaby, near Vancouver, British Columbia where his father retired in 1971 when Michael was 10. Michael attended several public schools during the time of his family's relocations. He dropped out of high school in the eleventh grade and never finished. (He earned his General Education Development (GED) certificate when he was in his 30's.) He did not attend college. Instead, he pursued an interest in acting.

At age 15, he starred in a Canadian Broadcasting Company sitcom entitled, "Leo and Me." In it, Michael played a 12-year old boy living with his Uncle Leo aboard a dilapidated yacht which Leo had won in a poker game.

In 1979, at age 18, Michael left Canada and moved to the United States where he settled in Los Angeles to advance his career as an actor. As is true with many young people who relocate to Hollywood because they dream of an acting career, Michael started out slowly suffering what he described as "humiliating and seemingly pointless auditions and routine rejections." But his luck changed. Between 1979 and 1980 he performed in 15 episodic roles on five television programs.

Against the odds and fortunately for him, Michael made his first film debut later in 1980 starring as Scott Larson in the film, "*Midnight Madness*." His second starring role was two years later in 1982 in the film, "*Class of 1984*." That same year he earned the lead role starring as Alex P. Keaton in the very popular television series, "*Family Ties*," which aired 176 episodes between 1982 and 1989. His popularity and reputation as a teen idol were enhanced further during that time by two blockbuster movie hits in 1985, "*Back to the Future*," and "*Teen Wolf*."

Michael met his future wife, Tracy Pollan, who was co-starring with him on the set of *Family Ties* in the role of his girlfriend. They were married in 1988 and have four children: son, Sam; twin daughters, Aquinnah and Schuyler; and daughter, Esme.

147

Over the course of his acting career, Michael performed in more than 40 television programs between 1977 and 2018, and starred in more than 35 films between 1980 and 2018. A truly gifted actor whose attitude, sentiments and personality fit the roles which he portrayed, Michael won a variety of awards to include five Primetime Emmy Awards, four Golden Globe Awards, two Screen Actors Guild Awards and one Grammy.

In 1991, at age 29, Michael received a confirmed diagnosis for Parkinson's disease. After a long period of reflection, he made a public disclosure about his status years later in 1998. He had battled symptoms daily, his condition had become progressively worse, and his ability to work and perform had been compromised by the disease. He wrote in 2009 that "Parkinson's had consumed my career, and, in a sense, had become my career."

Michael the actor, comedian and producer transitioned to Michael the activist and author. His wife would continue to be his greatest source of support. There had been nothing in his early career which had prepared him for a transition such as this and it was not easy. But he did have a huge circle of affluent, reputable and influential friends who were on hand to help.

To become a credible advocate for persons living with Parkinson's disease and to act on behalf of expanding research into the disease, Michael had to understand it better. He studied the literature, spoke with the medical and scientific professionals and participated, mostly anonymously, in internet support groups and chat room forums about Parkinson's disease. He learned from these activities that each person's experience with Parkinson's is different: onset, symptoms, attitudes, treatments, medications, dosages, side effects, therapies, support and environment. One advantage of Michael's notoriety and popularity was that, after his diagnosis became public, many people devoted and committed to research with the goal of finding a cure for this disease found an ally in him. They came from among support groups, medical professions, research institutions, lobbyists and foundations.

In 2000, before he started his new "day job" working to create and promote an organization or foundation dedicated to research and the quest for a cure, he took his family on a summer holiday to France. They resided in a villa not far from a town where France's most famous sporting tradition, the Tour de France, would pass. Days later, at a hotel in Paris, Michael learned that he and his family would share the hotel with famed cyclist and champion, Lance Armstrong, 10 years his junior, who not only had won the Tour de France but also had won his battle with testicular cancer.

Michael learned of the Lance Armstrong Foundation, created by someone as young as he, whose mission is to "inspire and empower cancer sufferers and their families under the

149

motto 'unity is strength, knowledge is power, and attitude is everything'." Substituting the words "Parkinson's patients" for "cancer sufferers" was motivational. Once of Lance's friends who had shipped some bicycles to Paris to ride with him during practices was Michael's friend from theater, stage and screen, Robin Williams. Robin would later would receive a diagnosis for Parkinson's disease dementia and dementia with Lewy bodies both of which dementias are characterized by abnormal deposits of Lewy bodies in the brain. Robin Williams died in 2014. Michael's time with his family in France, especially in Paris during the Tour de France celebrations, helped augment his desire to create a foundation where courage and hope were the motivators and accomplishment was the goal for finding a cure for Parkinson's disease.

Back in the United States Michael's friends, former co-workers, professional associates and others, many of whom had very deep pockets, from everywhere between Hollywood and Wall Street, worked to help raise money to create his foundation. One of the first "Michael J. Fox Foundation Planning" meetings took place in New York City in October 2000. By November 2000 the "Michael J. Fox Foundation for Parkinson's Research" was incorporated and certified as a not-for-profit organization. Its Chief Scientific Advisor was Dr. William Langston, the founder and Chief Executive Officer of the Parkinson's Institute. One of Michael's supporters at this time in New York City was actor, director and author Alan Alda, who received a confirmed diagnosis for Parkinson's disease this year in July 2018.

In March 2001, at a "Fight Night" annual fund-raiser for the Muhammad Ali Parkinson's Center in Phoenix, Arizona, Michael, at 5'5" and 130 pounds, and Muhammad, at 6'2" and 255 pounds, met and produced a joint public service announcement on behalf of Michael's new Foundation. The theme: "Together We Can Win This Fight."

Chapter 6, "Possible Causes," begins with one of Michael's observations with respect to the disease: "Genetics loads the gun and the environment pulls the trigger." His very first film, "Leo and Me," produced in 1976 when Michael was only 15, has become notorious for the fact that a disproportionate number of persons who supported that film as cast members and crew have received confirmed diagnoses for Parkinson's disease. Four of the 125 persons from the set include Michael, his director Mr. Donald Williams, a writer and a cameraman. This is one of the hundreds of factors which characterizes Parkinson's disease and which merits investigations and research of the types supported by Michael's Foundation.

The Michael J. Fox Foundation for Parkinson's Research continues its work to find a cure for Parkinson's disease primarily by funding research. Today, in 2019, it ranks first among non-profit organizations which fund research to find a cure.

Michael has related his story and promoted his work on a quest for a cure in three books. _Lucky Man: A Memoir_, published in 2002, describes his early life and acting career. Its focus is on the 10 years between his diagnosis in 1991 and the publication in 2002 during which he and his family adapted to the struggles associated with the disease, how his life had changed, and what he envisioned as opportunities for the future. His second book, _Always Looking Up: The Adventures of an Incurable Optimist_, published in 2009, tells again his personal and emotional responses to and actions after receiving his diagnosis and his decision, supported by his family, closest friends and professional associates, to work to build an organization which would support research to find a cure. The third book, _A Funny Thing Happened on the Way to the Future: Twists and Turns and Lessons Learned_, published one year later in 2010, uses materials from his first two books to highlight biographically his experiences and sentiments about his life, career, family, friends and future.

"In fact, Parkinson's has made me a better person, a better husband, father and overall human being." MJF

Pope John Paul II. (1920 - 2005)

"Remember one thing. Give without expecting to get back anything." John Paul II.

His Holiness Pope John Paul II, Bishop of Rome, Vicar of Jesus Christ, Primate of Italy, Patriarch of the West and leader of the billion-member Roman Catholic Church was born Karol Józef Wojtyla on May 18, 1920 in Wadowice, Poland. His father, Karol Wojtyla, was a tailor and later a soldier first in the Austrian Army and then in the Polish Army. His mother, Emilia Kaczorowska Wojtyla, was a homemaker. He was the second of two sons. His brother, Edmund, was 14 years his senior. The family of four lived in a three-room apartment in Wadowice.

The Wojtyla family was deeply religious. Young Karol's devotion to his faith and his respect for the teachings and traditions of the Catholic Church were guided and reinforced by the examples set by his parents in a country that was almost 90 percent Catholic.

He attended school in Wadowice where he sat in a classroom with as many as 60 other students. An exceptionally industrious student, his time in school was characterized by hard work and attention to detail, and was balanced by his interests and skills as a sportsman and athlete. He enjoyed hiking, soccer, skiing and swimming. His hometown at this time included a mix of Christians and Jews who were his neighbors, schoolmates, friends and competitors on the athletic fields.

In 1924, when Karol was only four, his older brother Edmund left home to study medicine at the Jagiellonian University in Kraków. Before

Edmund's graduation, his mother Emilia died in 1929 at age 45 following a long illness. A year later, in May 1930, Edmund was promoted to the position "Doctor of All Medical Sciences" at the Jagiellonian University. Sadly, just over two years later, Dr. Wojtyla died on December 4, 1932 at age 26 four days after contracting scarlet fever from a patient. Before he was 12, young Karol had suffered the loss of his mother and his brother writing later that "It was God's will." He remained at home together with his father who died in February 1941.

During his high school years, Karol continued to excel as a student and athlete and developed an interest in the arts, drama, music and poetry. He acted all four years during his high school education. He performed with his schoolmates at the Wadowice Theater Circle where he earned the admiration of his fellow thespians and their patrons as an accomplished actor with unique talents.

Shocking the world and beginning the start of the Second World War, the Nazis attacked Poland on September 1, 1939 when Karol was 19 and a student at Jagiellonian University. Throughout the terror of the Nazi occupation of Poland he continued his studies, athletics and acting until the Nazis clamped down on Polish society. They took over the government, closed his university and national places of worship, and arrested their enemies including Catholic clergy, Jews, intelligentsia and other perceived enemies of the State.

The future Pope witnessed the disappearance of his neighbors, friends, classmates, fellow clergy and thousands of others many of whom died in the big-city ghettos and in the concentration and extermination camps. His family's landlord for the three-room apartment in which he was raised was a Jew who perished with his wife and three daughters in the Belzec extermination camp in southeast Poland. Only an hour from his hometown of Wadowice was Poland's most infamous extermination camp Auschwitz. The largest of them all, more than one million people perished, 90 percent of whom were Jews.

In 1942, while Poland remained occupied by the Nazis, Karol was injured seriously. He was struck from the rear by a truck while walking home from his place of work. Knocked to the ground, he struck his head and lay there unconscious until, astonishingly, he was found by a German officer traveling in a military staff car. The officer had the future pope transported to a hospital where he was diagnosed with a concussion, treated and released. He recovered well enough to continue his studies as a seminarian and survive under the oppressive conditions of the occupation.

In Chapter 6, "Possible Causes," and earlier in this chapter in the narrative about Muhammad Ali, is a discussion about theories and studies concerning the effects of serious head injury and traumatic brain injury as possible triggers for Parkinson's disease. The accident and the concussion suffered by the seminarian may have been a factor contributing to the Parkinson's disease with which he was diagnosed 49 years later in 1991, 12 years after his investiture as the Pope.

But during this time, between 1942 at the height of the war and 1946 following the end of the war, seminarian Karol Wojtyla continued to study at a clandestine seminary for the priesthood whenever possible and wherever the architects of the Final Solution were not looking. The reality of the events of the Second World War and his devoutness as a seminarian during that time combined to propel him towards a vocation as a priest.

Karol Józef Wojtyla was ordained on All Saints Day, November 1, 1946 in Kraków. He celebrated his first Mass in a cathedral there the next day, All Souls Day. He left Poland for two years to study in Rome for a teacher's certificate. He returned to Poland in 1948 to serve as the pastor of a church in a village close to Kraków, so poor that it lacked both electricity and running water. In addition to his pastoral duties, he taught at the elementary schools in the parish. Seven months later he was back in Kraków serving in a larger church with more parishioners and a greater personal following. The threats to his ministry were from the communist governments installed by Stalin in the countries behind the Iron Curtain. Very familiar with the miseries inflicted by the Nazis, Father Wojtyla traveled, preached, lectured and organized among his countrymen working to keep the communists from repeating the evils of the Nazis. He was fearless.

His mentor, outspoken anticommunist Stefan Cardinal Wyszynski, was imprisoned and exiled by the government in 1953 for three years. Released as a hero, he nominated Father Wojtyla for elevation to Bishop. His consecration at age 38 took place on September 28, 1958, just shy of 12 years after being ordained a priest. Nine years later in 1967 Pope Paul VI elevated him to Cardinal. Following the deaths of two popes in 1978, the College of Cardinals elected Karol Cardinal Wojtyla to replace Pope John Paul I. John Paul II, the name chosen by the new pope out of respect for the three popes who served before him, assumed his duties as the Bishop of Rome on October 22, 1978. He was a very young and healthy 58 years old.

For 27 years between 1978 and his death in 2005, Pope John Paul II had a huge impact on the Catholic church and the world. In 1981, he survived an assassination attempt, later visiting his Muslim assailant in prison and forgiving him for his attempt to murder him. No one knows if this event was a second trigger for his Parkinson's disease.

Unlike any pope before him, John Paul II traveled the world during his 26-year pontificate to spread the word of the Gospel and to preach Church doctrine and his sentiments about the sanctity of life, equality, liberty, compassion, dignity, peace and love. He was the first pope ever to visit a mosque, to enter a synagogue and to establish diplomatic relations with Israel.

Together with such titans as Lech Walesa, Nobel Laureate and former President of Poland; Mikhail Gorbachev, former General Secretary of the Soviet Union; and, Ronald Reagan, former President of the United States, he helped bring about the collapse of communism in the former Soviet Union and East-bloc countries. After the Berlin Wall fell in November 1989, General Secretary Gorbachev stated that "the demise of the communist bloc would not have happened without John Paul."

John Paul II was named by *TIME* magazine as "Person of the Year" in 1994. He appeared 15 times on its cover.

In March 2006, a 120-page book entitled *"Lasciatemi Andare" ("Let Me Go"),* was published and contains comments by John Paul's personal physician, Dr. Renato Buzzonetti. They include a discussion about the assassination attempt and the diagnosis for Parkinson's disease and how they effected the life of the Pope. Dr. Buzzonetti confirms that the first symptoms of Parkinson's disease were diagnosed in 1991, and that the Vatican never formally acknowledged this until after his death. Except for what could be observed, the symptoms with which the Pope suffered never were disclosed by the Vatican. "Be not afraid" was his motto as he lived his faith and faced his death.

Pope John Paul II died in his private apartment in the Apostolic Palace of the Vatican on April 2, 2005. The cause of death was heart failure, circulatory collapse and septic shock. He died 46 days before his 85th birthday.

"The future starts today, not tomorrow." Pope John Paul II.

Deborah Jane Trimmer. (1921 - 2007)

"I'd rather drop dead in my tracks one day than end up in a wheelchair in some nursing home watching interminable replays of The King and I." DJK

Deborah Jane Trimmer was born on September 30, 1921 in Helensburgh, Scotland. Her father, Arthur Charles Trimmer was an aviator, civil engineer and naval architect who served in the military in Europe during World War I. He died of tuberculosis in 1937 at age 43. Her mother, Kathleen Rose Smale Trimmer, was a homemaker. Deborah had one younger brother, Edmund, five years her junior. In 1939, she changed her name to Deborah Jane Kerr following the recommendation by her agent at the London Theater Group that it would enhance her career as an actress. Kerr was the family name of her maternal grandmother.

As a child she was shy and sensitive. She also was very self-disciplined and obedient enjoying what she recalled as a normal childhood for a young girl living with her brother and parents at home before the war in Europe. She had flat feet and was mildly afflicted with scoliosis which she said dashed her dreams to be a ballet dancer. But she exercised daily to improve her posture and walk, including spending time lying on the floor to keep her back straight. She read and was absorbed by the stage and film magazines which she obtained and sensed that she always wanted to be a performer.

The happiness which she enjoyed with her family was interrupted when she was sent away in 1933 at age 12 to a boarding school more than 100 miles from her home and family. Her natural shyness made her a target for teasing and abuse by other girls at the school. But she endured. A few years later her fortune changed when her aunt, a radio actress and manager for a drama school, offered her a position. She blossomed as a performer and moved to London in 1939 at age 18. While she worked there, she suffered with the Londoners enduring the air raids and bombings by the Nazis. She found great joy and satisfaction entertaining the Allied troops during the war.

In 1945, after the war ended, she met and married a British Air Force officer who distinguished himself with the Royal Air Force as a combat pilot during the war. After a seven-month courtship she married former Squadron Leader Anthony Bartley on November 29, 1945. In 1946 they moved to Los Angeles where Deborah would continue to advance her successful career as an actress. Their first daughter, Melanie Jane, was born the next year on December 27, 1947. Their second daughter, Francesca Ann, was born four years later on December 20, 1951.

The children remember doting parents and as happy a childhood experience that the Hollywood environment could offer any child whose parent or parents moved frequently between home and wherever the next motion picture set was located. If Deborah's success as an actress had an effect on her children it had a greater and opposite effect on her husband. Their marriage faltered, then disintegrated. They divorced in 1959.

That same year she met Hollywood screenwriter Peter Viertel, born to Jewish parents in Dresden, Germany in 1920. They fled the Brown Shirts and other aspiring Nazis for California in 1928. Peter was graduated from Dartmouth in 1941, enlisted in the Marine Corps after the Japanese sneak attack on Pearl Harbor, fought against those fanatics in the Pacific, then served in Europe where his German language skills were exceptionally valuable. Peter and Deborah married in 1960 in Klosters, Switzerland where they lived together in the resort mountain town.

Deborah's career spanned six decades. Her persona as an actress was characterized by her femininity, sensitivity, radiant beauty, elegant style and enormous passion for the roles she played: everything between nuns and nymphomaniacs. She played her first role in 1940 as a cigarette girl in the film,

"*Contraband.*" She played her last role in 1986 as "Emma Harte" in the film, "*Hold the Dream.*"

In the 56 years between those two films she starred in 52 other films. She earned six Academy Award nominations for her performances in "*Edward, My Son*," (1949, Best Actress); "*From Here to Eternity*," (1953, Best Actress); "*The King and I*," (1956, Best Actress); "*Heaven Knows, Mr. Allison*," (1957, Best Actress); "*Separate Tables*," (1958, Best Actress); and, "*The Sundowners*," (1960, Best Actress). She never won an Oscar. Over the years she would tell her family, friends and others, "Always a bridesmaid, never a bride."

But in 1994, when she was 72 years old, living with Parkinson's disease, and in obvious physical decline, The Academy of Motion Picture Arts and Sciences, awarded Deborah Kerr an "Honorary Career Oscar." The Oscar was inscribed "To an artist of impeccable grace and beauty whose motion picture career has always stood for perfection, discipline and elegance." True to character, she stood on stage, unassisted at a microphone, and told the assembled audience in a clear, distinct voice that "You have made my life truly a happy one. I thank you from bottom of my heart."

In 1997 she was made a Commander of the Order of British Empire by Queen Elizabeth II.

Well after her retirement and while secure in her home in the Swiss Alpine resort town of Klosters, Deborah granted a very limited number of interviews to select persons. She focused on her career, her life in retirement and provided only a few details about her health and living with Parkinson's disease. In 1999, when she was 78, she said that her health began to fail when she was in her 70's. She confirmed a diagnosis for Parkinson's disease in 1994 when she was 73 and she immediately began a regimen of medications which had helped to keep her in good health.

As is true for almost all persons who receive a diagnosis and who start a regimen of medications, there were unsettling side effects and the medications and dosages had to be changed. She credited the medications for improving her mobility but remained bothered that her occasional incapacitation made her irritable. Other manifest symptoms included tremors, difficulty walking, freezing and problems with balance. She was frustrated with the knowledge that people who recognized her as Deborah Kerr, star of stage and screen, and who may have seen her stagger as she walked and slur her words as she spoke, would think that she may have been drunk. Obviously an easy target for the contemptible paparazzi, incidents such as this justified her desire to live and enjoy her retirement as a private person.

Deborah Kerr died in the village of Botesdale, Suffolk County, England on October 16, 2007. She was 86. Her husband of 47 years, Peter Viertel, died three weeks later.

"There is a way around everything, good or bad, if you are smart enough." DJK

Janet Wood Reno (1938 – 2016)

"I made the decision long ago that to be afraid would be to diminish my life." JWR

Janet Wood Reno was born on July 31, 1938 in Miami, Florida. Her father, Henry Olaf Reno, was a career reporter for the *Miami Herald.* Her mother, Janice Wallace Wood Reno, also was a journalist, writing for the *Miami News.* She had three younger siblings, two brothers, Mark and Robert, and a sister, Maggy.

Ms. Reno attended public schools in Miami-Dade County, Florida. She was graduated from Cornell University with a degree in Chemistry in 1960, and from Harvard Law School in 1963. After graduation from Harvard, she returned to Miami and worked as an attorney for eight years through 1971.

Still residing in the Miami area, she transitioned to working for local and state government organizations. In 1978, the governor of Florida appointed her the first woman County Attorney in the state. She served in Dade County. Also in 1978 she won an election as State Attorney General, an office which she held through four more successful elections.

In 1993, President William Jefferson Clinton nominated her as his Attorney General. On March 11, 1993, the Senate confirmed Ms. Reno by a vote of 98 to 0. When she was sworn in the next day, she became the first female United States Attorney General. Another first!

Her career as Attorney General was compromised by several serious controversies. She made decisions and directed actions which not only threatened American civil liberties but also resulted in the state-sponsored murder of 103 American citizens, the arrest of a police officer falsely accused of committing a terrorist action at the 1996 Olympics, and the deportation of a six-year old Cuban refugee from freedom with his family in America to oppression with the communists back in Cuba. But, serving in an administration in which her boss also was surrounded by controversy and eventually impeached by the Senate, her decisions and her actions faded relatively quickly from the front pages and the public's memory.

On November 16, 1995 Ms. Reno announced that, at the end of October, she had received a confirmed diagnosis for Parkinson's disease. She was 57 years old, slightly younger than the average age of 60 for persons who receive such a diagnosis. At that time, she stated that her symptoms were mild, that she considered herself to be in good health, and that she planned to remain in office and continue her duties.

Her announcement took place almost as a

matter of routine at her weekly news conference. She told those assembled that, during the summer of 1995, she had noticed her left hand shaking. When the shaking did not go away, she became concerned and consulted a doctor. She informed the President and senior members of his administration and her staff about the diagnosis.

The initial and obvious symptom was the tremor. A combination of the drugs carbidopa and levodopa had succeeded in controlling the shaking. At the news conference she added that, "I feel fine now. I do not feel as if I have any impairment." Her neurologist, Dr. Jonathan Pincus, at the Georgetown University Medical Center, stated that "nothing about the disorder she has should impair her capacity to do her job."

But two years before the diagnosis, as the nation's top law enforcement official, she ordered the raid on the Branch Davidian compound in Waco, Texas which killed 86 adults and 17 children. She took full responsibility for the raid and apologized. Only six months after her diagnosis she again was the United States' principal law enforcement officer who falsely accused police officer Richard Jewell of committing a terrorist act at the 1996 Summer Olympics in Atlanta, Georgia. She offered her second official apology. Then, three years after her diagnosis, she made the decision to remove six-year old Elian Gonzalez, whose mother had drowned bringing him from Cuba to the United States, and to return him to Cuba. For this action she did not apologize.

Janet Wood Reno died among her family at home in Miami, Florida on November 7, 2016. She was 78.

"Just remember, strength and courage. Given that you'll never lose."

Margaret Bourke-White (1904 - 1971)

"To understand another human being you must gain some insight into the conditions which made him who he is." M-BW

Margaret White was born on June 14, 1904 in The Bronx, New York. Her father, Joseph White, son of a Jewish immigrant from Poland, was a naturalist, engineer and inventor. Her mother, Minnie Bourke, daughter of a Catholic immigrant from Ireland, was a homemaker. She had two siblings, a sister Ruth, older by three years, and a brother Roger, younger by seven years. The children grew up first in New York and then in New Jersey before attending college.

In 1922, when Margaret was 18, she enrolled in Columbia University but dropped out after only one semester. Next, she attended the University of Michigan, where she met and married Everett Chapman, an electrical engineering student. She transferred with him to study together at Purdue University. But the marriage was not a happy one, and the couple divorced after two years in 1926. They had no children. After the divorce, Margaret decided to change her name, adding her mother's maiden name "Bourke" together with her childhood family name, "White." Throughout the rest of her life she would be known as Margaret Bourke-White.

Following Purdue, she enrolled in Western Reserve University and finally Cornell University from which she was graduated in 1927 with a Bachelor of Arts Degree. Of the three White children, only Margaret bounced through five universities in five years. Her brother Roger wrote in his autobiography that his and his sisters' educations were provided "thanks to a rich uncle's financing." How very fortunate, especially in Margaret's case.

Cameras and photography were her hobbies. She created a stunning collection of photographs of the universities, the communities which supported them and the people within them. In 1928, she moved from Ithaca, New York to Cleveland, Ohio where she opened a commercial photography studio. She expanded her interests to architectural and industrial photography perhaps because both her father and her brother were engineers and industrialists.

There, Margaret, her photographs and her skills as a photographer came to the attention of Henry Luce who, at age 24, had published the first issue of *Time* magazine in March 1923 together with three fellow dropout classmates from Yale University. In 1929, Margaret was hired by Henry Luce as the first photographer for his new magazine, *Fortune*. He helped open up doors for her as a photographer, especially through another of his nationally famous publications, *LIFE* magazine. Luce hired Margaret in 1936 as one of the four original staff photographers for *LIFE.* She would achieve acclaim as the woman who took *LIFE's* first cover photograph. She remained working at *LIFE* until 1957.

Margaret enjoyed an outstanding career as a photographer and photojournalist earning a reputation as a professional young woman as distinctive as aviator Amelia Earhart and astrophysicist-astronaut Sally Ride. She toured the world with a camera with the same vigor and spirit as General George Patton who told reporters that he was "touring Europe with an army." Both were unstoppable!

In 1939, she met and married her second husband, American novelist Erskine Caldwell. Together they became a part of history as it happened.

Before World War II she toured Germany, Austria and Czechoslovakia as the Nazi war machine was flexing its muscles. During the war, she became America's first female war correspondent who was permitted access to combat zones. "Maggie the Indestructible" was the only foreign photographer in Moscow when the Nazis attacked the Soviet Union in June 1941. During the battle of Moscow, she survived raids by the Luftwaffe and bombardments by the Wehrmacht. At that time, her husband was working as a foreign correspondent in the Ukraine. The chaos and confusion of the war and the conflicts which arose from different careers and assignments resulted in Margaret's divorce from Erskine in 1942. As was true in her first marriage, the couple had no children.

In December 1942, she was a passenger aboard the British troop transport, the SS Strathallan, which was torpedoed and sunk by the Nazis in the Mediterranean. She shared a lifeboat with General Eisenhower's secretary, Kay Summersby.

"Maggie the Indestructible" first sensed the onset of Parkinson's disease from symptoms which she experienced in 1952 while she was returning home from the Korean war. She was 48 years old and now a victim of Early Onset Parkinson's. She did not disclose her condition to her friends and coworkers. Instead, she tried by herself to manage her early symptoms of left-side pain and tremor in her arm and leg. She did what she thought would help her manage her symptoms. She began a regimen of exercise, work and movement. To maintain her mobility, she walked regularly and learned to dance the Tango. She forced her muscles to work to maintain her posture, gait and balance while she moved. To control the involuntary contractions of her fingers closing to form a fist she rolled pieces of newspaper into balls which she squeezed and released. At that time in 1952, medications were not available and nothing such as Deep Brain Stimulation had been conceived.

Two years later, when she was only 50, her symptoms became more severe and she was forced to limit her work and travel. She had difficulties with tremors and mobility which were not responding to her regimen of exercise and physical therapy. She had brain surgery in 1959 when she was 55, and again two years later in 1961 when she was 57. The surgeries helped to calm her tremors but they also greatly affected her speech.

In 1963, after the publication of her autobiography, "*Portrait of Myself*," she became increasingly debilitated and reclusive. In the summer of 1971, when Margaret was 67, and 19 years after her first experience with the symptoms of Parkinson's disease, she fell. The fall was so severe that she broke several ribs. While hospitalized, she was unable to perform any therapy to aid in her recovery. She lingered, became increasingly debilitated, and could not speak beyond a whisper. "Maggie the Indestructible" had met her match.

Margaret Bourke-White died in the hospital in Stamford, Connecticut on August 27, 1971. She was 67.

"To know Parkinson's, you must know awkwardness, anxiety, and near-panic." M-BW

"Ask not what your family can do for you. Ask what you can do for your family."

James Vincent Pelosi. (January 21, 1961, President John F. Kennedy's inauguration.)

13. THE KENNEDY FAMILY

This chapter has nothing to do with Parkinson's disease as it has been described in the first 12 chapters. It has everything to do with family values, and what I consider to be an unacceptable way to care for a family member who is born with a handicap and becomes severely disabled.

The family I chose to provide as an example of poor performance caring is the Kennedy family: father Joseph P. Kennedy, mother Rose Fitzgerald Kennedy and eight of their nine children. The one child who is excluded is the third child, Rose Marie (Rosemary) Kennedy, the family's oldest daughter, handicapped her entire life, and whose experiences because of her handicap are the subject of this chapter's narrative.

Rosemary was born in September 1918; diagnosed as a toddler at about age two with a mental disability; lobotomized in 1941; and sent away from the family for her education, rehabilitation and basic life care until she died in 2005. Rosemary was considered an embarrassment to her high-profile businessman and politician father who demanded perfection from his wife and family.

I never heard of Rosemary Kennedy until sometime in 1960 when her older brother, John Fitzgerald Kennedy, was campaigning as the Democratic Party's candidate for President of the United States. In Chapter 1, "Introduction," I wrote that I grew up on a street where "there were 26 families with 48 school-age children." Eleven of those families were Catholic and all of them had at least two children. In 1960, there was an interest among many Catholics nationally to elect the country's first Catholic president. The Catholic Church took no position on the issue.

My father, who was a volunteer within the community for the "Get Out the Vote" effort by the local County Voting Board, hosted a function for our neighbors in the huge basement of our home. I listened to the conversations among our neighbors and my parents' friends while sitting on the top step of the stairs, at the ready, when summoned, to help refresh the food and drinks and empty the trash. I was nine years old. The strongest sentiment that I remember having heard had nothing to do with the opposing Party platforms, the candidates' experiences and qualifications, or their religious preferences. It had almost everything to do with the fact that the Democratic candidate and his family had mistreated one of their own, their third child Rosemary, who was cloistered after her tragic birth defect was discovered, then sent away and basically abandoned after her lobotomy. In 1960, while the Kennedy family was living the life of the rich and famous in their east coast estates and summer retreats, Rosemary, since 1949, had been sent to live among the nuns at St. Coletta's in Jefferson, Wisconsin, more than 1,100 miles away from them. The nuns, not the family, cared for the lobotomized Kennedy daughter for the remainder of her life.

In the basement that evening almost 60 years ago, the shared sentiment I remember hearing from the mothers was, "How could any mother do something like that to one of her children – especially with all their money?"

To support their own families at home, nine of the 11 neighborhood fathers worked more than one job. My dad worked three: one during the week at a bank; one on Friday nights at the Belmont Racetrack counting money and proving the tills; and one as a business consultant serving as the financial advisor and accountant for the owners of a local shopping mall. His fourth job, as an officer in the United States Air Force Reserve, he never thought of as a job. Flying aircraft was fun, not work.

So, who was this Kennedy family? What made them unique among other American families? Most importantly, who was Rose Marie Kennedy, and what does her life experience represent to the Parkinson's community?

Joseph Patrick Kennedy Sr. was born in Boston, Massachusetts in 1888, the eldest of five Kennedy children. He was graduated from Harvard University in 1912 at age 24 and started a career in business and finance. In 1913, at age 25, he held the title of "Bank President." After an eight-year courtship, he married his beau, Rose Fitzgerald, in 1914. The Kennedy couple had nine children between July 25, 1915 and February 22, 1932: Joseph Patrick (Joe Jr.) in 1915; John Fitzgerald (Jack) in 1917; Rose Marie (Rosemary) in 1918; Kathleen Agnes (Kick) in 1920; Eunice Mary in 1921; Patricia Helen (Pat) in 1924; Robert Francis (Bobby) in 1925; Jean Ann in 1928; and, Edward Moore (Ted) in 1932. Joe Kennedy's early successes as a businessman, bank President, and commodities, real estate and stocks investor provided the wealth which supported him and his large family as well as a nurse, governess and domestic help at the family home, and their support staff when they traveled.

Their third child and first daughter, Rose Marie, was born on Friday the 13th, in September 1918. When Mother Rose went into labor at the Kennedy home, the nurse who was present attempted to contact her obstetrician in Boston. There had been a doctor present in the Kennedy family home when the family's first two children were born.

However, the nurse was not able to contact the doctor immediately. He was moving throughout Boston treating people who were stricken by the Spanish flu pandemic of 1918 which infected one-third of the world's population and killed approximately 670,000 Americans. No one in the Kennedy family had been infected.

Rose's nurse had been trained to deliver babies; however, she also had been trained to wait for a doctor to make the delivery. Rose's contractions became more severe. She was not able to control the natural impulse to deliver the baby. The nurse's appeals to Rose to try to resist the contractions and hold her legs together once the baby had entered the birth canal failed. Then, the nurse made the flawed decision to reach into the birth canal and hold the baby's head as an effort to keep the baby inside her mother until the doctor arrived. This effort lasted approximately two hours with disastrous consequences for the baby. The doctor finally arrived and made the delivery. In all appearances, the baby seemed as healthy as the first two children. She was named Rose Marie after her maternal grandmother.

However, it soon became apparent that the lack of oxygen during the time that the nurse had held the baby's head inside the birth canal, had resulted in slowed development, physical impairment and brain damage. Perhaps six months after Rosemary's first birthday, when Mother Rose was pregnant with her fourth child, she noticed that Rosemary was not progressing as a toddler at the pace and with the skills that she had observed in her first two children. But Rose dismissed the slower development as only a condition natural to the differences between boys and girls.

To complicate matters further for the family, Rose, who knew that her husband had a reputation as a "ladies' man," suspected him of having an affair. While still very much pregnant and close to delivery, she moved out of the family home and left Joe Sr., along with the nursemaids and staff, to care for the three children. Her suspicions were correct. Soon her husband would be known as a womanizer, having affairs with a variety of attractive women including actress Gloria Swanson, 11 years his junior. Meeting the crisis with a renewed dedication to her Catholic faith, Rose returned home where she gave birth to her second daughter, Kathleen, on February 20, 1920. Rosemary was 17 months old.

About this time, both Joe Sr. and Rose became acutely aware of Rosemary's impairments. She had difficulty holding pencils or crayons when drawing or scribbling. She was uncoordinated and sometimes imbalanced when playing children's games. Her parents noticed that where other children at or close to her age were progressing easily with childhood tasks and play, their daughter was having difficulty and was slower to make progress.

Eunice, the family's fifth child and third daughter, was born on July 10, 1921.

In 1923, at age five, Rosemary began kindergarten at the Edward Devotion School, the same public school which her brothers Joe Jr. and Jack had attended. The teachers and staff who knew her brothers recognized that she was not as intellectually gifted as the boys. Only a kindergarten student, she, surprisingly, was evaluated as "deficient." This is an incredibly severe evaluation given the minimal events and activities in any kindergarten class; given a child's first time away from everything familiar to her at her home; and, given the uniqueness and levels of development of the other students who are strangers to each other. Mother Rose became Rosemary's coach, trying to help her master the tasks which she found difficult.

Rose's efforts were not rewarded and did not help Rosemary to meet school standards. In 1924, her teachers refused to promote her to the first grade. They told Rose that her daughter "was retarded." Rosemary repeated kindergarten. She took an Intelligence Quotient (IQ) test, a new educational tool in the 1920's, administered by the public-school system. Rose was told that her daughter's "IQ was low." The score is not known. Rosemary was promoted out of kindergarten after her repeating her second year.

Patricia, the family's sixth child and fourth daughter was born on May 6, 1924. Brother Bobby, the family's seventh child and third son, was born 18 months later on November 20, 1925. That year, Papa Joe, who owned several movie theaters in New England, purchased a motion picture production company in California, further expanding his investments portfolio and increasing the family fortune.

In 1925, Rosemary started the first grade and ended in 1926 with same level of unacceptable achievement as she did after her first year in kindergarten. She was forced to repeat the first grade. Her playmates and the other girls her age were entering the fourth grade.

Following the birth of her sister Jean Ann on February 20th (the same day as her sister Kathleen) in 1928, the Kennedy clan now numbered eight: five girls and three boys. The family relocated to support Papa Joe's work and the continual need for larger homes for his expanding family and their at-home support staff.

Rosemary was bounced among local public and boarding schools. Her parents, determined to find a school which was acceptable to them and also suitable for Rosemary's special needs, were very reluctant to describe to the administrators and educators the full extent of her disabilities as they knew them. Their expectations were that she meet the standards achieved by the other Kennedy family children, and that she be treated in the same way as her fellow students. Regardless of how her parents tried to disguise the reality of her impairments, much about Rosemary was obvious. The three "R's": Reading, wRiting and aRithmetic were a struggle for her. She had problems with her ability to write and spell, and the manner by which she wrote and formed her letters were evidence of severe learning disabilities. She remained poorly coordinated and unskilled at games and sports. The family knew well that, as Rosemary continued to age, the differences between her and her peers were becoming increasingly more evident.

In the fall of 1929, before the crash of the stock market, Rosemary, now 11, was sent out of state to Pennsylvania and enrolled in a private school for children with special needs. Although the relocation was, at first, difficult for her, she adjusted. Rosemary made sufficient progress at the end of her first year for the staff to report favorably to her parents about her progress. However, they did comment that they considered her educational difficulties to be related directly to a lack of confidence and low self-esteem which made her frequently frustrated and irritable.

The Kennedy family's final child, Edward Moore, was born on February 22, 1932. Joe Sr. and Rose became parents of nine children: five girls and four boys.

In 1934, Rosemary, at 16, had been enrolled in two more private schools, a total of three schools in only five years. Each relocation, and each adaption to a new school in a new location with new staff and new students was an emotional challenge for her. Rosemary always was slow to adjust. At no time and in no school was she ever able to attain the social skills and the educational achievements that would meet her parents' expectations.

That same year, President Franklin Roosevelt appointed Joe Sr. as chairman of the Securities and Exchange Commission. Three years later, in 1937, he received a second presidential appointment as chairman of the Maritime Commission, an important and highly-visible position given the threat of war in Europe at the time when Hitler and the Nazis were becoming increasingly belligerent. Only a year later in 1938, President Roosevelt appointed him ambassador to the Court of Saint James in England, the first time that an American Irish Catholic was selected to serve in this position within the Protestant realm. Given all the prestige, glamor and international attention associated with his role as ambassador, Rosemary's status, at age 20, created a huge threat to what the parents wanted for the public's perception of the Kennedy family as intelligent, charming, graceful, and seemingly, the perfect American Catholic family.

Rosemary did well during the family's relocation to London. She was the most beautiful of the five Kennedy daughters, attracting much attention, especially that of the young men of status in London. She remained at a distance from the public and the press unless she were escorted closely, usually by her sister Kathleen or another family member. At the annual presentation at court, Mother Rose, Rosemary and sister Kathleen were presented to King George VI and Queen Elizabeth. But even though Rosemary had practiced the presentation for weeks, she tripped, but did not fall, in front of the King and Queen. While others may have been embarrassed by the faux pas, it later was very obvious that Rosemary was not. She danced the night away with a variety of titled suitors.

In 1939, before the Nazi attack on Poland and the start of World War II on September 1, Rosemary was a student at a private Catholic school, the Covenant of the Assumption, located not far from the American embassy. The environment and regimen of instruction and tutoring as needed worked well for Rosemary's special circumstances. After the war began, all the Kennedy children returned to the United States. Rosemary and her parents remained in England. After France and Belgium surrendered and were occupied by the Nazis in May 1940, Rosemary returned to the states with friends of the family. Shortly afterward, London and Embassy Row became a prime target for Luftwaffe bombings.

Back in the United States, Rosemary once more was sheltered and cloistered by her parents who continued to shield her disability from almost everyone outside the family, with the exceptions of a few very close friends and the staff that was hired to support the family household. At 22, Rosemary's striking beauty attracted the attention of many men. Her parents knew that Rosemary would not have the mental capacity to sense their ultimate intentions and that she would be vulnerable to their intimate pursuits.

In 1940 and '41, Rosemary continued to be bounced in and out of schools in the northeast. As usual, no school was suitable for her parents, and Rosemary's attitude, lack of focus and actions, bordering on combativeness, were not helpful.

What would prove to be a disastrous event for Rosemary, happened not long after Joe Sr., initially in consultation with his wife, began to investigate the possibility of surgery to correct Rosemary's disabilities. For more than 20 years, the Kennedys had sought relief for Rosemary and her condition from professionals in a variety of medical, psychological, and educational research specialties. Joe Sr. had read and heard about brain surgery conducted to improve very serious mental-health disorders.

In 1941, there had been articles about lobotomy surgery published in *The Saturday Evening Post*, *The Richmond Dispatch* and *The Journal of the American Medical Association.* Although there was hope that this new type of surgery could help resolve the impairments of the mentally disabled, the early literature cautioned that this type of surgery, known as a pre-frontal lobotomy, still was in the pioneering stages. It had been performed in the United States for less than three years. Further research still was needed; not enough surgeries had been performed (fewer than 100 patients to date); and some mental health professionals had criticized the surgery as unscientific and dangerous, citing the serious evidence of significant problems and unsatisfactory results.

Mother Rose enlisted her daughter Kathleen's support to help gather the information necessary for her parents to make a decision. Kathleen responded and strongly advised her mother against proceeding with the surgery, telling her, "Mother, this is nothing that we want done for Rosie."

It is not known if there were any consultation between Joe Sr. and his wife or any discussion that may have included the older children. But sometime in the fall of 1941, Joe Sr. made the decision to have the surgery performed on Rosemary. He did not inform his wife nor any of the children. Given Rosemary's mental capacity, it seems reasonable to assume that she, too, was not informed, but no one knows.

In November 1941, Rosemary was admitted to George Washington University Hospital in Washington, D.C. The doctors who performed the surgery were Dr. Walter Freeman, a neurologist, psychiatrist and professor at George Washington University, but not a surgeon, and Dr. James Watts, a neurosurgeon. The Freeman-Watts team had performed the first lobotomy surgery in the United States only five years earlier in 1936. At that time in late 1941, they had performed only about 80 such surgeries.

Prior to the operation, Rosemary's head was

shaved and she lost one of her physical attributes which made her so very beautiful. In the operating room, Rosemary was strapped to a table and given a local anesthetic to numb her brain. While she remained wide awake, Dr. Freeman directed Dr. Watts, the surgeon, to drill two holes into each side of Rosemary's skull near the temples. Rosemary would have sensed the drilling sounds much the same way as a dental patient senses a dentist drilling a tooth. When the drilling finished, Dr. Watts made an incision through the two holes into each side of her brain. Next, a tool, similar in appearance to a butter knife, was used to scrape away brain matter at the frontal lobes. Still wide awake, Rosemary was directed to speak, recite and sing so that the doctors could evaluate to what degree they were affecting the brain. The scraping and cutting continued until Rosemary became delirious and stopped speaking.

The doctors paused then stopped the operation and made an evaluation. After only a couple of hours, the doctors decided that the operation had gone terribly wrong. The consequences were horrifying. Rosemary was unable to walk or talk. She was nearly completely disabled. She never regained the ability to use fully her arms and her legs. One arm and one leg were entirely dysfunctional; the other arm and leg barely functioned. She was paralyzed on her left side.

Rosemary was left with the mental abilities of a toddler, unable to form a sentence or to follow simple directions. Only 23, she never again would be able to care for herself in any capacity. How traumatic an event was this bungled operation? Shocked, sickened and traumatized by the events of the operation, the attending nurse quit nursing completely.

While Rosemary continued to linger in the George Washington University Hospital, Mother Rose, shortly after the operation, wrote a family letter on December 5, 1941 to all of the other children. She did not mention Rosemary. For the next 20 years Mother Rose never again mentioned her first-born daughter and third child to anyone in any of her letters. More reprehensible for a mother is the fact that there is no one's recollection and no evidence that Rose ever visited her severely disabled daughter for more than 20 years.

Later in December 1941, Rosemary was relocated to Craig House, licensed in 1919 as the country's first private psychiatric institution. It was located in Beacon, New York, approximately 50 miles north of New York City on the Hudson River. She lived there in a one-bedroom, one-bath cottage until 1949. Joe Sr. quickly relocated Rosemary after allegations surfaced that she may have been sexually abused. During her seven years at Craig House, only Joe Sr., but not her mother nor any of her eight siblings visited.

This time she was moved to St. Coletta's School, a Catholic facility for the mentally disabled in Jefferson, Wisconsin. On-site at the school, Joe Sr. funded the construction of a one-story brick cottage where Rosemary would live for almost 60 years more than 1,000 miles away from her family.

Rose Marie Kennedy died at Fort Atkinson Memorial Hospital in Wisconsin with her sisters Eunice, Jean and Pat and her brother Ted at her bedside on January 7, 2005. She was 86.

On January 21, 1961, after dinner together as a family, we retreated to the living room to watch the evening news. Most networks aired an extended broadcast which highlighted the inauguration of John Fitzgerald Kennedy. In his inauguration speech, President Kennedy made the comment, "Ask not what your country can do for you. Ask what you can do for your country."

The inauguration was almost 20 years after his sister Rosemary's lobotomy.

In 1955, my father, with three children born in 1951, '52 and '53, started work as a volunteer and ex-officio Board of Directors member for the "St Giles in the Fields" institution for children built in 1903 in Garden City, New York, only five miles from our home. Its mission was to provide care, treatment and medical research for disabled children.

Given the Kennedy family's celebrity status, and his work at St. Giles, my father knew enough about the many details concerning the

Kennedy family's "missing child" to criticize the family's behavior toward their disabled child and sibling.

He told us what he knew about Rosemary. After he mimicked the line from the President's speech and said, "Ask not what your family can do for you. Ask what you can do for your family," he explained to us three children, then ages seven, eight and nine and all enrolled in Catholic elementary school, that the situation with Rosemary was a "good example of bad behavior." I know that all of us were too young to understand what he was trying to teach us. But what I remember most distinctly is his comment, "With all their money and all their property, could his (President Kennedy) father not have built the same cottage in Hyannis Port or in Palm Beach, and kept his entire family together?"

I know now, after 18 years of research about Parkinson's disease and after 10 years of caring for my mother in my home while she lived with Parkinson's, the value of unrequited love when caring for someone who is severely disabled. A family member's touch, embrace, the sound of his voice, and the awareness of the acts being performed lovingly to do the things he cannot do for himself, all are life-sustaining highs for someone living with Parkinson's. This could have been the case for Rosemary had she not been cast aside by her parents and her family.

"Oh, James, I don't know why the Good Lord gave this to me."

Dorothy Rinderknecht Pelosi.

14. DOROTHY, MY MOTHER.

The Early Years as a Child.

My mother, Dorothy Muriel Pelosi, was born on May 20, 1924 in Elmhurst, Queens, New York. Her father, Charles Rinderknecht, born in 1896, worked two jobs as a deliveryman, one providing milk and the other providing coal. They were delivered by means of horse-drawn vehicles. Her mother, Elsie Cosgrove Rinderknecht, born in 1899, was a homemaker. My mother had one sibling, a sister, Katherine, older by four years. The family was practicing Catholics. When my mother made her Confirmation at age 10, she took the name Hyacinth.

The girls had a difficult childhood. Their father left home very early in the morning, seven days a week, to begin his delivery routes and finished in mid-to-late morning.

Often there were complaints about the delivery service, and he was forced to rectify those complaints before he received his daily pay and returned home. By then, any of the many pubs in the neighborhood would have been open, and he may have visited at least one for a nip or two or ten.

Their mother was an alcoholic. She died in 1930 at age 29 of a brain aneurysm when her daughter Katherine (Kate) was just shy of 10 years old and my mother just shy of six. My mother told me that she remembered nothing about her mother: not her appearance, not the sound of her voice, nothing about their homelife, and nothing that they ever may have done together. All her life she and her sister remained loving daughters exceptionally dedicated to their father who died in 1967.

The small homes in Elmhurst which my grandfather was able to afford had four rooms: one bedroom, a small living room, kitchen and bathroom. The bedroom was furnished with one full-size bed in which my grandfather slept. In the living room was one three-seat sofa on which his sister slept after the death of his wife. My Aunt Kate slept on a two-seat swing set kept within the home and brought outside on the porch when the weather was nice. My mother slept in an oversized, stuffed chair. She told me that, after she and her sister arrived home from school, they would try to sneak naps on their father's bed. Usually they woke to feel the sting of his belt on their legs when he came home after a long, hard day at work and, frequently, some time at a pub.

The kitchen table was a recycled card table for which there were four folding chairs. Two were at the table and two were stored in a corner to make room within the apartment. My Aunt Betty did not cook. She took most of her meals at work. My mother never had canned beans in our home when I was a child. She told me that for supper her father usually opened two cans of beans and served one can to each girl, often cold and with a spoon stuck in the center of the can. Over the course of our lives together, I never saw my mother eat beans anywhere at any time.

The stock market had crashed less than six months before Grandma Elsie's death. Thousands of people in the area were without work. Anti-social behavior and crimes of all types rose significantly.

Elsie Rinderknecht's obituary was published in the local paper. While the now three-person family was at the funeral Mass and cemetery, thieves broke into the home and stole everything of value including small furnishings and appliances, photos, mementos, most of the clothing, all the kitchenware: pots, pans, dishes, utensils, linens, and toys, if there were any. Their father's only sister, Elizabeth Werner, born in 1882, moved in to the home and performed all the duties of a surrogate mother and companion to her brother.

When the girls still were in grade school,

but old enough to wake to an alarm clock, attend to their hygiene, find something for breakfast, dress and walk to school, Elizabeth moved out to a small apartment close by and took a job as a clerk at Stern's department store in New York City. Aunt Kate then slept on the three-seat sofa; my mother traded the overstuffed chair for a place on the two-seater swing.

The money Aunt Betty earned helped everyone, especially on those all-too-many occasions when my grandfather drank away the rent money and the family was dispossessed. As a child, I remember my mother telling me and my sisters that when she and her sister came home from school, on at least three or four occasions they would find their furniture and possessions at the curb and a neighbor waiting to escort them to wherever some kindly person had found shelter for them. Their father lost a day of work and occasionally his job when he took off the day after they were dispossessed to relocate the furniture and possessions. The girls' lives never were routine or predictable.

In addition to his sister Elizabeth, my grandfather had three younger brothers. One brother, William (Willie), lived with his wife, son and two daughters on Long Island, not far from his widowed brother and his two motherless nieces. Uncle Willie's two daughters were close in age to my mother and aunt, only four and six years younger. On the weekends and whenever their Uncle Willie was able, he would travel into Elmhurst and bring the girls home with him for the weekend and occasional holidays. In his family's country-setting home in Wantagh, the girls could escape the crowded apartment, play with their cousins outdoors in their large yard, neighboring fields and parks, eat full and sufficient home-cooked meals, and sleep in real beds. As a child, my mother told me that, had I not been named James after my father and his father, I would have been named William after this very loving uncle who died three years after I was born.

The youngest of my grandfather's siblings was his brother, Fred, who was born in 1906 and who died at the age of 106 in 2012. The Rinderknecht parents could not afford to raise five children. At a very young age, Fred was given up to Catholic Charities and raised in an orphanage ("home" as he referred to it), while he awaited adoption. At about age 12, he ran away and found work with room and board on a farm in upstate New York. He ran away from two farms because he was mistreated, finally remaining on the third farm where he raised his family and ended up owning for about 80 years.

When Fred was 25 and newly-married, my grandfather was convicted of a crime for which he received a long prison sentence. But there was no one to care for his two daughters and a deal was made on their behalf. My grandfather would serve his sentence beginning in early summer when his daughters finished school for the year, and would be released in late summer in time to support them at home before the start of the new school year. During those summers, the girls were bused to upstate New York to live with my Uncle Fred and his wife, Ollie, and their new baby Laura born in 1934. (There was only 10 years difference between my mother and her Aunt Ollie, and 10 years difference between my mother and her first cousin Laura.) My grandfather's sentence was commuted for hardship and compassionate reasons after his daughters had endured this routine for six or seven summers: no one in the family today remembers exactly.

My mother told me that she feared the long-distance bus ride alone with her sister and surrounded by strangers; the long wait at the bus stop some place remote and unknown to them in upstate New York in all types of weather; the strangeness of a large farmhouse with no indoor toilet – the outhouse was 20 yards from the rear door and lacked electricity; the vastness of 400 acres of farmland with huge plow horses and milking cows; and, no playmates other than each other. But she did say that her aunt and uncle were exceptionally kind and benevolent; the meals were wonderful and the snacks frequent; the dogs, cats, kittens were everywhere and their antics were comical. Family again became her refuge.

Given the circumstances of their difficult life at home and away during several summers, both my mother and aunt, rather surprisingly, were very good students. As the older sibling, my aunt was the trailblazer and used her academic prowess to help my mother when she started grade school. I know that my mother enjoyed high school, perhaps not so much for the academics, especially French language class, but more for the socialization with other maturing girls and boys as she came of age.

Aunt Kate was graduated from Newtown High School in June 1938. Following graduation, she worked as a sales clerk in a department store in New York City. Later she was promoted to Assistant Buyer in the women's clothing department. Her boss was absent from work one day and my aunt had to travel to her home in Brooklyn to have some papers signed. There she met her future husband, John Daspro.

My mother was 17 and a junior in high school when the Empire of Japan conducted its sneak attack on Pearl Harbor on December 7, 1941. Many boys from Newtown High School in Elmhurst left school before graduating in order to join the military. Most of these boys were seniors about to graduate in six months; many were my mother's junior-year classmates. But, because of the war, my mother's class was graduated earlier in January instead of in June 1943. In her year Newtown High School yearbook, there are photos and captions for the 233 boys in her class: 18 had enlisted and did not graduate. Following their name and photograph, 83 of the other 215 boys who did graduate had the name of a branch of service after the word, "Destination:" (Destination: Marines; Destination: Army; Destination: Navy."

My mother's experiences sometimes mirrored my own. I am a Vietnam-era veteran. That war had been raging since I started high school in 1965. The surprise Tet offensive in January 1968 swelled the number of Americans serving in Vietnam dramatically. Still in high school, I knew seniors and juniors who either dropped out of school before graduation to serve in the military or who waited until after their graduation to join.

One day, after I came home from school, I mentioned this about my schoolmates to my mother. She told me that much the same had happened in her high school after the attack at Pearl Harbor, and about her high school classmates during World War II. She said that the first boy who ever walked her home from school, the first boy who ever carried her books home from school, the first boy who ever held her hand for any reason, the first boy who ever asked her out on a date, the first boy who ever brought her to a dance, and the first boy who ever gave her a kiss all joined the military.

She wrote letters to them, and they wrote back to her from their training and duty locations and from their combat arenas. Some sent her souvenirs. She showed me a bracelet from a Marine in combat at Tarawa, a miniature set of airborne jump wings, a patch from a Marine Corps division, hand-carved crucifixes, and small wooden-bead bracelets. All six of these boys, four of whom were Marines, were killed by the Japanese in combat in the Pacific. She kept all their letters and all the keepsakes that they sent to her. Until she died, 69 years after the attack on Pearl Harbor and 65 years after the Japanese surrender, my mother never would ride in a Japanese-built automobile: not by herself, not with another family member, not with a friend, never.

My mother was graduated from Newtown High School in January 1943. She was hired as a clerk and secretary at Chase National Bank in Queens, New York. My father had been hired by the same bank working at what was called a "rat clerk" sorting cancelled checks after his graduation from Flushing High School in June 1941. Born on December 11, 1923, he was only 17 years old when the Japanese attacked Pearl Harbor. My grandmother, a widow, would not sign his enlistment papers to allow him to join the military. He waited four days after the attack and then joined the Army. He had the promise of a job with Chase Bank when he returned after the war.

In great physical shape and with perfect vision he was selected to train as a pilot in the Army Air Corps. He was commissioned a Second Lieutenant after successfully completing his flight training. In 1942, his first assignment was as an instructor pilot within the United States and Rio Hato Air Base in Panama. In 1943, he was assigned to combat duty in Europe ahead of and in support of the Allied invasion at Normandy, France on June 6, 1944. After the war ended, he returned home to Flushing. He donned his bemedaled Army Air

Corps dress uniform with its Captain's insignia of rank and walked into Chase Bank. He did not ask about the earlier promise of his job back after he returned. He had no interest to return as a rat clerk.

At the bank he saw the woman whom he would marry and she saw him. They spoke briefly at their first meeting, but longer in the early evening after she finished work and they had their first date.

After Aunt Kate married in July 1943, my mother then had the three-seat sofa on which to sleep. She told her children that until she married our father in January 1950, she never slept in a bed of her own. When she married my father, she was 25 years old. He was 26.

The Later Years as a Wife and Mother.

After my parents married, my mother was a stay-at-home wife living in a small, two-bedroom, fourth-floor walkup apartment in Flushing, not far from the Chase Bank where my father was re-hired, not as a rat clerk but as an Assistant Manager.

My mother miscarried her first child in the spring of 1950 and her fifth child in the spring of 1959. But between those misfortunes, I was born on July 10, 1951. My sister Kathy came around 363 days later on July 8, 1952. When my mother became pregnant with her third child in February 1953, my parents concluded that the fourth-floor apartment was too small and too burdensome for my mother. My parents bought a home on Long Island where we four and then my sister Janet, born on November 1, 1953, in Flushing Hospital, came to live.

Within this narrative, in this book's first chapter, "*Introduction*," there are three short paragraphs which describe my family's new neighborhood. My father commuted from our home town by train into the New York City area until he retired in 1981. My mother remained a stay-at-home mom until my sister Janet began high school in 1967. Then she took a job at Doubleday Book Company in Garden City, New York as an accounting clerk. The wife of one of my father's coworkers at Chase Bank, with whom my mother was a close friend, found her a position with her at Equitable Life Insurance Company also in Garden City.

My sister Janet married in February 1975, and moved into an apartment in a beach town about nine miles from our home. Kathy married in May 1978 and remained in our hometown less than two miles from where we were raised and where my parents still lived. She worked as a flight attendant for American Airlines. She flew on a pass once to Berlin to visit me during Thanksgiving week in 1976 when I was assigned there with the Army.

She became a mother in 1980 and again in 1981, the year of my father's retirement. My parents assumed the role most grandparents enjoy (?) today, that of on-call baby sitters and care providers for their grandchildren. After the birth of her second child Kathy left her job with the airlines.

The Later Years.

Very early on in the marriage, troubles developed between Kathy and her spouse. They divorced before the children started school and Kathy obtained custody of their two very young children. Again, my parents tried to enjoy their life in retirement including vacationing to Florida where they had purchased a home. But always there were reasons why they were needed to care for their grandchildren. My mother helped with grocery shopping, made meals, did the laundry, walked the children to and from school, helped them with their homework, cared for them when their parents were absent.

Over time, after Kathy had been institutionalized for drug- and alcohol-related problems and had received a diagnosis as bipolar manic-depressive, my parents assumed vastly expanded roles in the care of their grandchildren. I helped when I was assigned at the United Nations for nine months. My parents helped Kathy and the children relocate to Florida to a home within five miles of theirs and continued their care and support. Later, Janet, as godmother, obtained custody of the children when they were in their early teens, and Kathy could not function as a mother.

My father died of cancer in January 1996, two days before my parents 46th wedding anniversary. My mother wrote in her journal, "I was proud to be his wife."

200

My mother and I were at his bedside daily with my father from the last time that he was admitted to the hospital until he died. I brought my mother home in the evenings when it seemed as if my father was asleep and would sleep through the night. Every evening I returned and stayed with him overnight in an oversized chair in his room. If he woke during the night, I helped him with whatever he needed.

One time, when we were alone, he said to me, "James, promise me that you'll take care of your mother." I assured him that I would. I knew that when he used the words, "you'll take care of your mother," he meant that I would be her sole care provider for her when necessary, not some hired stranger in some type of facility.

Next, he said to me, "I want be cremated, and I want you to keep the ashes. When something happens to your mother, I want our ashes to be mixed and be buried together."

Given the events of my mother's youth before she was married, (described above at length), the loss of her lifetime companion was devastating. Although she did not manifest any obvious signs of depression, she started to slip. After my father's death, I drove the 90 miles between our homes weekly or bi-monthly and helped my mother with everything related to maintaining her health and her home. Frequently, I returned with her to my home in Melbourne where she would visit for two weeks or more. I think that we were good company for each other. She made new friends with some of the retirees in my neighborhood.

In January 2000, I was reassigned from the NASA Kennedy Space Center and Patrick Air Force Base to the Johnson Space Center in Houston, Texas. One day in late spring of 2000, when my mother was caring for the children at their home, they came home to find her lying prone on the kitchen floor. She either fell and broke her hip or she broke her hip and then fell. She was 75 years old.

She did not respond to the physical therapy at a rehabilitation facility after she was discharged from the hospital following the surgery to repair her broken hip. She was readmitted to the hospital where X-rays revealed that the surgery was flawed: there was a gap between the implanted pins and her bones; the hip still was broken. The second surgery required an additional fracture to repair her hip. Her response to the physical therapy following the second operation was much worse than after the first operation. Perhaps because she feared falling or perhaps she no longer was physically able, she never walked again.

At the end of the spring and through the summer my sisters cared for our mother at Janet's apartment. Janet worked as a grade-school teacher and was home full-time during the summer recess to manage our mother's care. Kathy rented a unit in the same apartment complex. At that time, I purchased a large, four-bedroom home in Clear Lake only four miles from the Space Center. There I worked with building contractors to make improvements and revisions to the structure of the home anticipating that I would welcome my mother who no longer would be able to live alone.

The contractors built a concrete ramp leading into the rear of the home; removed the original door frames and added new, wider doors which would accommodate the passage of a wheelchair; added safety grab bars in all the bathrooms; installed elevated toilets for ease of movement from and to a wheelchair; and, replaced the thick carpet and pad in the bedrooms and hallways with a thinner and smoother carpet.

Within three miles of my home, in the same professional medical complex where I brought my two dogs, Sheba, a black Labrador and Gizmo, a Lhasa Apso, to a veterinarian, there was a medical doctor and a dentist. The medical doctor was female. She agreed to accept my mother as a new patient. At the dentist's office, I spoke first with his wife who worked as his receptionist and appointment scheduler. While we were speaking, I noticed a diploma on the wall identical to one which I had earned. Dr. Charles Whatton is a 1969 graduate of the United States Military Academy. He was graduated four years ahead of me. He, too, agreed to accept my mother as a new patient. He and his wife, Jennifer, and I and my mother had a very wonderful relationship. Finding that complex clearly was meant to be.

Two doors down from Dr. Whatton's office was a beauty parlor. I spoke first with the scheduler and next with a beautician, Ms. Tammy Lord. I told Tammy that sometime soon I would bring my disabled, wheelchair-bound mother to live with me. I asked her if she would be able to provide a "wash and set" service for her. I told her that I would transfer her between the wheelchair and the chairs at the wash basin and styling area. She said, "Sure, no problem." Within a week or two, I met Tammy again at the local American Legion Post where I was a member and where she worked a second job as a bartender.

At the "Acknowledgements" section within this text is my recognition of the Whatton family's and Tammy's love and long-term support for my mother and me.

Near the end of the summer, I made arrangements with my sisters to travel to Florida over the long Labor Day weekend and return my mother with me to Texas. Before then, I wrote an ad for a home health-care aide. I published it on Craigslist, and also distributed it as a flyer which I posted at the three hospitals and several nursing and assisted care facilities locally in Clear Lake. (A copy of that ad is included in the text at Appendix 4, "Ad For Home Health Care Aide.")

On the first day that the ad appeared on Craigslist I received 46 responses. At one response, which contained a very impressive resume, the writer asked, "Mr. Pelosi, please call me."

I did. We introduced ourselves and then I said: "I have had more than 40 responses in the first six hours that the ad appeared. Do you have any idea why so many people might be interested in this position?"

Emma answered, "Mister Pelosi, this is something special. You are asking for someone to care for one person in the privacy of a single-family home in a very nice neighborhood. And you are offering to pay more money with more paid time off – no weekend or holiday duty – than we get in a facility where get paid less money, have less time off, and have to care for between six and eight people of all sizes with all sorts of medical issues. I'm sure that every person who reads your ad will respond."

I think that Emma was correct. Within eight hours of posting there were more than 70 responses which overwhelmed me. I deleted the ad. I answered every response and interviewed five people, including Emma. I asked each of the five candidates whom I interviewed that, if she were not selected, would she be willing to return in the future if I should need her as a replacement aide or for supplemental help. Without exception, everyone said, "Yes." I hired Emma, and asked her to meet me on Tuesday morning after Labor Day at the home at 8 a.m., after Labor Day.

The Final Years Together Again.

The flight between Florida and Texas was not difficult. Airport security and United Airlines were very helpful. Our seats at the bulkhead provided the extra space to maneuver my mother from and to her wheelchair.

After we were airborne, the aircraft had reached cruising altitude, and the "coffee, tea or me" service had ended, my mother fell asleep. I said a prayer, a very rare activity for me, and asked God, "Please keep me healthy throughout the time that I am caring for Mom. After that, do what you want. Amen." He did.

The ride from the airport to my home was just at an hour. After we arrived, Sheba and Gizmo, who had known my mother for six years before their relocation with me nine months earlier, rushed to greet her.

I spent the remainder of our first day together in Texas getting her settled. But after we arrived, and while the weather was still warm, I took her on a walking tour of the neighborhood. I pushed the wheelchair while Sheba and Gizmo walked close beside or behind us. Ordinarily they were fairly responsive to voice commands, unless there were other animals in the area. Any neighbors' pets that they recognized usually were inspected then ignored. Any strange animal, especially a squirrel within striking range, sent them on a sprinting frenzy.

This type of activity served multiple purposes. My mother enjoyed watching Sheba and

Gizmo agitate each other, and they got their exercise beyond their regular walks. She got to be outdoors and break up the rather-sterile routine indoors. She met our neighbors and made new friends. These would be the folks on whom I might have to rely in the event of an unexpected difficulty or an emergency. One of my mother's greatest joys was watching small children at play. Our home was within a neighborhood filled with children. Our street with 14 homes hosted school-age children in nine of them. The grade school was less than 300 yards away, easy biking or walking distance for most of the children without any roads to cross.

I took off the Tuesday following Labor Day to meet Emma, describe her duties, and walk her through the routine. After she arrived, I re-introduced her to my mother, (she met her the first time during her interview at my home), and, for the second time, we toured the home and the property. I provided her an information sheet which described my mother's status and listed her duties which I explained. Then I demonstrated part of the daily routine as I performed it.

I told Emma that I woke my mother every morning at 5 a.m. and transported her to the toilet to clean her and refresh her clothing if necessary. I added that I had made the same effort five hours earlier at midnight trying to ensure that she would be clean and in fresh bedclothes as she slept. Every morning, my mother would be clean, refreshed and back in bed by 5:30 a.m. After I fed and walked the dogs, prepared the breakfast, and wrote any instructions, I would leave for work at 7:40 a.m. to start not later than 8 a.m. My mother still would be asleep and alone in the home for 20 minutes until Emma arrived. I asked Emma to look in on her immediately after she arrived and to call me. Usually, all she had to tell me was that everything was fine in the house and that my mother was asleep. I would remind Emma to wake her and start the day's routine between 8:30 a.m. and 8:45 a.m.

I demonstrated how I transferred my mother from her wheelchair to the toilet, attended to her hygiene and changed her overnight clothing. From there we moved to the kitchen where the table had been set for breakfast. At this time, my mother still was able to eat and drink without assistance. Morning medications were part of the breakfast. After she finished, I cleared the table, hand-washed the few dishes and let my mother dry them. That activity enabled her to focus on the chore, coordinate her eye and hand movements, and move her arms, hands and fingers. (A second similar chore, which also required her to coordinate her eye and hand movements and to use her hands and fingers, was to fold the small items from the weekly laundry.)

From the kitchen I transported her to the living room and transferred her to a sofa where she sat and then reclined supported by a pillow. While she watched the morning news, I showed Emma the contents of her clothing closets, dresser and jewelry boxes. The dogs loyally stayed beside my mother who, bored by the television noise, took a short nap.

When she woke, I demonstrated the routine when I returned home from work at the noon hour. I moved my mother from the living room to bathroom where I ran the water in the jacuzzi tub to give her a bath. Then I undressed her and moved the wheelchair perpendicular to the tub. I stripped to my briefs; stood in the tub; lifted my mother's legs over the rim of the tub; then picked her from the wheelchair and seated her gently in the warm bubbling water.

While she soaked, I put on a pair of gym shorts and T-shirt and took the dogs for a quick walk, leaving them to explore in the large, fenced-in yard after we returned. In the kitchen, I placed a casserole dish containing a pre-cooked meal (protein source, starch and vegetables) in the oven to warm. Then I went to attend to my mother in the bathtub. I undressed again, turned off the jacuzzi, and draped a large bath towel on the wheelchair. I got into the tub, lifted and turned my mother and lowered her on to the wheelchair. After I got out of the tub, I covered her with a second bath towel and dried her. I told Emma that this was the time that I would dress to return to work.

I dressed my mother while the lunch meal warmed. When I was finished, we moved to the kitchen. There it would become Emma's task to serve the meal for my mother (and for herself if she desired). Following lunch, the routine would be the same as after breakfast: Emma would clear the table and hand-wash the dishes. My mother would dry them.

In the early afternoon, if the weather were pleasant, Emma would walk my mother for a 30-to-60-minute stroll. Often this was at the time that the school children were returning home. At other times they sat outside on the backyard patio talking, or Emma reading and my mother watching the dogs or napping.

In adverse weather, my mother enjoyed resting on the sofa in front of the wide-screen television and watching what we called, "The Old Movie Channel," (Turner Classic Movies) where she could view films that she knew and enjoyed. In the television cabinet was a large collection of DVD's that included musicals, such as *West Side Story*, *Gigi*, and *Hello Dolly*, and films, such as *Casablanca*, *Gone With The Wind*, and *An Affair to Remember*, which kept her attention.

Saturday evenings, after Mass and dinner, she also enjoyed viewing two comedies presented by the BBC: *Are You Being Served?* and *Keeping Up Appearances*. Both of these shows made her laugh, even those which were repeated and which she had seen. Laughter certainly may be the best medicine.

Finally, I told Emma that I would call her daily at or around 5 p.m. when I would be leaving work. I would be home less than 15 minutes after calling. After I arrived, and

After Emma described her day to me, she would be free to depart.

In the early evenings, I would take my mother, Sheba and Gizmo for a ride just over one mile from our home to the University of Houston, Clear Lake. The campus is more than 525 acres and home to a variety of wildlife including alligators, wild turkeys, bobcats, and whitetail deer. The deer population was between 50 and 100 and, although wild, very tolerant of the student, faculty and tourist traffic which passed by them. My mother enjoyed watching them roam and feed. Sheba and Gizmo were eager to be set loose to start a chase.

Once back at home, I fed Sheba and Gizmo and prepared and served dinner. My mother took her last medication with her meal. We finished around 7 p.m., and the start of the daily Turner Classic Movie, most of which were rarely more than two hours long. After the movie, I tended to my mother's hygiene and dressed her for bed. She would be in bed not later than 9:30 p.m. and asleep almost immediately.

I slept in the same room with her so I could hear her if she woke. I went to bed at 10:30 p.m. waking at midnight for the regular check-and-change which took less than 15 minutes. I woke again at 5 a.m. for the morning check-and-change after which my own day began.

Emma worked diligently, faithfully and caringly for us for three months. Then she gave me notice that she would have to leave.

Her younger sister was in the terminal stages of cancer and she was needed to provide care for her.

During the time that Emma helped me care for my mother, I tried to understand more fully what her experience was like after she left the rehabilitation facility and went to live with my sister Janet in her two-bedroom apartment. In one room, my mother slept in a Medicare-provided hospital bed. At night and whenever someone was not in the room with her, the side security bars were raised for her safety. But the first time I saw my mother in that type of bed she said to me, "James, please get me out of here. I feel as if I'm in a jail." My sisters were doing their best, so I said nothing to them. I told her that I had bought a home in Texas, that I was having the home renovated to support her living there, and that I would return shortly (it took almost four months) to bring her to Texas to live with me.

The aide whom my sisters selected to care for my mother came from Haiti. I never asked my sisters how they determined that she merited the position. She was a large woman. When I saw her hug my mother when they greeted each other, or when I saw her embrace my mother to transport her it appeared as if the life were being squeezed out of her. I saw my mother grimace slightly, but I never heard her complain.

The aide had the benefit of bringing her two

young, grade-school-age boys to work with her when they were not in school. Although they may have been company for my mother, in the small apartment their presence seemed overwhelming. When one boy sat on my mother's lap in the wheelchair I sensed that it was not a comfortable experience for her. The aide cooked Haitian food which my mother never before had eaten. Given my mother's experiences in her youth, she had no one to teach her and very little time to learn how to cook. As children, we never ate spicy foods of any kind.

The aide was paid a salary of $500. a week. At that time, in Haiti the average annual income was $504. That salary was paid by my sister from funds in my mother's account. Each month, the salary alone exceeded my mother's combined income from Social Security and her widow's pension by $600. Her income was reduced further by the purchase of care-maintenance supplies such as adult diapers, wet wipes, gloves, and household items such as food and cosmetics. During her six-month residence, my mother's finances decreased by $7,000. At that rate, given my mother's longevity (an additional 10 years) her savings would have come close to depletion.

I described previously for the purpose of alerting family members that the costs of in-home care for a person living with Parkinson's disease have the potential to be devasting in the long term if sensible budgeting and strict spending standards are not maintained. It was

213

my experience that caring for my mother at

home for 10 years cost me personally only an average of $12,000. to $15,000. a year, which is far less expensive than the costs of care within some professional facilities.

When I left my mother in January 2000 to start work in Texas she could walk, drive a car, shop, cook, clean and maintain her health and hygiene. She weighed between 125 and 130 pounds maximum. When I saw her during her first hospitalization, I knew that she had lost some weight. When I saw her again four months later, she had lost even more weight. After she arrived with me in Texas, she weighed only 108 pounds.

Before we left my sister's home for Texas, she provided me mother's medical records and documentation which indicated diagnoses for Parkinson's disease, osteoporosis, depression and mild dementia. She also provided me bottles of pills.

As a cadet at the Military Academy, throughout my time in the military, and most of my life including now, I have been a history buff. My father, his brother, their cousins and their schoolmates from their neighborhoods all served in World War II. The experiences of anyone who had served in that war fascinated me. My first assignment in the military was in Berlin. Frequently, I toured Germany and Europe. In three years, I visited nine of the former Nazi concentration camps.

I learned that Holocaust survivors and former prisoners in Europe, Russia and the Pacific, who had been starved during their imprisonment, changed dramatically. Beyond the physical impairments they also suffered mentally and emotionally. Following their liberation or release, many did not know their names or their ages, who their family members were, how long they had been a prisoner, or where they had lived before capture or arrest, deportation and imprisonment. One major reason for this debility was the lack of any fat in their diets. The brain uses fat to process information.

After I assumed the care for my mother, underweight and overmedicated, I resorted to the techniques used to help revive Holocaust survivors and restore their health if possible. First, I added fat to her diet. That included a one-scoop dish of Texas' famous and especially tasty Blue Bell ice cream at lunch and again at dinner. Next, I threw out all the medications prescribed for depression and dementia. After I saw my mother improve, I described the improvements to my sister, a vegetarian who does not eat anything "that ever had or would have had a face." She complained to me that, "Mom's cholesterol is high and she needs to avoid fat to keep her cholesterol low."

My response was, "What for?"

In 2000, she already had exceeded her life expectancy of 60 by 16 years! She had a confirmed diagnosis for Parkinson's disease which, although not a killer disease in itself, is a life-limiting disease. She enjoyed eating foods that tasted good, and most tasty foods, especially desserts such as pie and ice cream, contain fat.

For the 10 years that she lived with me, she was hospitalized only once for a urinary tract infection and a second time to have her gall bladder removed. Those were the only two times that she ever lost weight again. She never had the flu. She never was sick. She never complained of pain. As she aged, she tended to tire more easily and her waking hours became shorter; however, she had boundless energy whenever she was participating in something that she truly enjoyed. She had annual physicals, annual flu and pneumonia shots, quarterly dental examinations and teeth cleanings. No tweaks ever were made by her doctor or her neurologist to her Parkinson's medication: carbidopa-levodopa.

Several years ago, a close family member in his 40's suffered a stroke. To the best of our knowledge there never was any history of stroke on our side of the family. As a teenager, he worked in an ice cream store and, perhaps as a result of that experience, shunned eating ice cream for about 30 years. Following the stroke and after he had been released from the hospital, he finished the therapy to help restore his body to its previous functionality. An MRI taken at that time revealed two substantial black areas of his brain that had 'died' from the stroke.

Sometime later he developed a sudden urge for ice cream. He told me that he probably ate more than he should have, having gained what he considered was an unacceptable amount of weight. But the ice cream worked wonders to help restore his functionality. Having reviewed this chapter of the book prior to its publication, he called to tell me his story. I am very grateful for his interest, this contribution and his support.

At our home, my mother's weight stabilized between 120 and 125 pounds. I considered any weight below 118 pounds to be an indicator that something might be wrong, and any weight at or below 115 pounds as a certainty that something was wrong. She may have weighed between 115 and 118 pounds when she died, certainly a result of not consuming food for 10 days and liquids for four days before her death.

There were no issues of dementia. She recognized and communicated with our family members and her long-term friends who spoke to her in person or by telephone, with her home health care aides, with her doctor, dentist and beautician, with our neighbors whom she saw regularly, and with the astronauts and NASA employees whom she knew from NASA-related functions and from holiday and card parties I hosted in my home. At those parties, she sat in the living room and shared their company. When the aide would tell her that it was 10 p.m. and time for bed, she always refused to leave the party. She would remind me of my great-grandmother's comments when her daughter would try to coax her to bed, "Not now, Mary. There is plenty of time for sleep in the grave." She was alert the entire time of any party. The aide would go home and I would put my mother to bed around midnight after the last guest departed.

I know what brought my mother back to life after her hospitalizations, attempts at rehabilitation, and living undernourished and overmedicated. I know why she enjoyed a happy life for 10 years as a person living with Parkinson's. Some of the reasons I've written above. Other reasons are still to follow.

Despite issues which existed between my sisters and me, most of which concerned the status of our mother, we remained compatible.

During the Christmas season I always took two weeks' vacation from work. The aides also earned a two-week paid vacation. When Janet was off for what her school called "Winter Recess," and Kathy was between jobs, my sisters would travel to Texas to spend Christmas with us. It always was an enjoyable time, and my mother thoroughly loved their company. At night, one sister would share the Queen-size bed with her mother; the second would sleep in what was my bed. I slept in a guest bedroom. Together, my sisters resolved any issues overnight with my mother. Usually, there were none.

During the summer, I frequently traveled to Europe on government business, while working primarily with Italian universities and science and engineering companies to design, integrate and manifest experiments for demonstration by the astronauts on the Space Shuttle or International Space Station. Before I departed from Orlando to Rome, I would pack my mother, Sheba, Gizmo and all the travel essentials for the 1200-mile, two-day drive to Florida. Sheba and Gizmo would stay with Helen in Melbourne. My mother would stay with my sisters at Janet's home.

My sisters once told me, after they had seen my vehicle loaded with me and my mother, the dogs and as-needed bags with snacks and hygiene supplies piled up inside the vehicle, and the portable toilet and wheelchair strapped to a bicycle rack at the back of it, that we looked like the *Beverly Hillbillies* on their trip between Tennessee and California. They were right. The hillbillies probably had an easier drive.

We would make a rest stop for all of us every four hours, and a stop for food and fuel every eight hours. On the stops at a Rest Area along I-10 traveling east, I would park in a space designated for the handicapped.

I would open the windows about half-way and leave my mother alone while I took Sheba and Gizmo for a walk where the vehicle and my mother remained in sight. When we returned, I gave them water each in their own bowls, and a treat or two, and let them jump back into the rear seat of the car.

Then I would remove the wheelchair from the

bicycle rack and take my mother and her Tote bag of personal hygiene supplies from the car. While the dogs watched from the half-open windows, we walked to the restrooms. If the one handicapped facility were not available, I would bring my mother into the ladies' room. Before we entered, I would knock, then announce, "Man entering with disabled female." I knocked and made the announcement two or three times before entering. Any woman who may have been agitated by my presence usually settled down when she saw me bring my mother into the handicapped stall. When we were finished, we returned to the car. As we came into view, Sheba and Gizmo acted as if we had been gone for a month.

I always booked a hotel room for the one overnight stop which accepted dogs, had a ground-floor handicapped room with two beds, and a restaurant within the hotel. After we arrived, my mother, Sheba and Gizmo remained in the car while I registered. Then I took the dogs for a walk and brought them to the room. I left them there with their supper and water and retrieved my mother and only the luggage needed for overnight and the following morning.

In the room, I tended to my mother's hygiene while Sheba and Gizmo fought at each other's food dish. (There was not enough room to separate them with the distance that they were used to then eating at home in Texas.) They stayed in the room while my mother and I went to dinner. Following dinner, and after I had

220

my mother cleaned, dressed and in bed watching television, I took Sheba and Gizmo for their final walk of the day. Gizmo slept in the bed with my mother. Sheba slept on the floor next to my bed, the same sleeping arrangement as if we were in Texas.

The next morning, after I performed the usual 5 a.m. check-and-change for my mother and returned her to bed, I took the dogs for a walk and returned. By 10 a.m., we had finished breakfast in the room, checked out and departed. We arrived in Melbourne around 8 p.m. Helen walked and spoiled Sheba and Gizmo while I settled my mother in Helen's home and managed the luggage.

Sheba and Gizmo stayed with Helen when I brought my mother to Janet's home. Two weeks later, I reversed the direction of travel from Florida back to Texas with much of the travel routine on the return trip identical to the routine on the outbound trip.

I enjoyed my time at work in Italy. The girls enjoyed their time with their mother. It was hard for me to separate Helen from Sheba and Gizmo.

In July 2000, Colonel Ronald Garan, United States Air Force, was selected as a pilot by NASA. He would train be an astronaut and fly a Space Shuttle. He and his wife, Carmel, and their three sons, Ronnie, Joseph and Jake, relocated to Houston and moved into the home next-door to ours. They are a wonderful family and were fabulous neighbors. Over the years that we were neighbors in Clear Lake, we spent much time together, the Garan family frequently hosting us at their home on holidays and special occasions.

In 2002, my mother and I attended the NASA ceremony recognizing Ron's transition from Astronaut Candidate to a member of NASA's newest class of astronauts. In May 2008, we traveled to the Kennedy Space Center to view the launch of Space Shuttle Discovery and Ron's first flight as a Mission Specialist.

Carmel had served with the Air Force as an Emergency Room nurse. I am embarrassed to write that I may have abused our friendship when I took advantage of her skills to ask her for advice with medical issues relating to my mother. Carmel always was available to help us. After my mother's two hospitalizations, she visited and helped me and the aides to modify her daily routine until she regained her strength and vitality.

At the time of the publication of this book, Carmel's mother, too, is a person living with Parkinson's disease. Carmel frequently travels long distance from her home in Tucson, Arizona to Pennsylvania to help her sisters and family care for their mother in her home.

The Garans moved five miles away to the town of Nassau Bay into a home on the water. They sold their home to the Arnold family. Ricky Arnold had been selected by NASA as an Educator Astronaut in May 2004. He moved next-door with his wife, Eloise, and their two daughters, Carrie and Jessie.

Ricky made his transition from Astronaut Candidate to a member of NASA's newest class of astronauts in February 2006. My mother and I attended his ceremony. We also traveled to Florida in March 2009 to view Ricky's launch aboard Space Shuttle Discovery, (the same Shuttle on which Ron Garan had flown one year earlier).

The Arnold family was as much a blessing for us to have as neighbors as was the Garan family. NASA has done well recruiting the best and the brightest to serve as astronauts. Everyone in these two families was a great source of happiness for us.

Mary replaced Emma as mother's second home health care aide. She was one of several children born to an Air Force family whose primary stateside duty locations were in the southern United States. She had earned a high school diploma and had taken additional courses in technical subjects and the liberal arts at specialized schools and junior colleges.

After high school, Mary had the wanderlust, and traveled through the southern states along the Gulf of Mexico mostly in Alabama, Mississippi, Louisiana and Texas. I asked her how she supported herself.

She told me, "Mister Pelosi, I slip-slided my way through them states until my lawyer told me I'd probably be declared 'persona non grata' and end up in jail."

I had no idea what she meant.

Mary had discovered that she could find her way to any of several nationally-known department, home improvement, or grocery stores and locate the water fountain. When she thought no one was looking, she'd take a drink of water and let more water spill out onto the floor. Then she'd take a short 10-second walk in a semi-circle, passing by the same water fountain and pretend to slip. She'd fall down, cry out and wait. The system did the rest to provide her support. Mary would receive more-than-sufficient "compensation for injuries" that would hold her over until her funds ran low and she had to find a different store in which to "work."

She told me that one of her sisters had asked her how she managed to pay rent, keep a functioning automobile, buy groceries, go to the movies and socialize all without a regular job. Mary's answered, "It's easy. I'll show you."

Mary explained the routine to her sister and demonstrated the technique in one store doing everything except slipping and falling. Then they went together to a second store. Everything went well, except that her sister slipped and fell for real! A large woman, she twisted her ankle, fractured her tibia (the small bone in the leg below the knee cap), fractured her wrist, and broke two fingers.

Mary added that she said to her sister as she tried to pick her up, "Lizzy, you dumba**! How can you be so stupid? You weren't supposed to fall for real." Lizzy was hospitalized, went through rehab, relocated with another sister, and spent all the compensation money before she was able to walk and return to her former job.

Finally, Mary told me that one of her lawyers told her that her name and ID had come up so often in injury-related compensation claims, that it would not be long before she was caught and probably imprisoned. She said, "I decided to find Jesus," which she did.

Mary found a religious institution to sponsor her education. Being the daughter of a retired senior Air Force member (who was a committee member and spokesperson in his church), having a high school education and a clean record, she was accepted, trained and ordained a minister.

But Mary told me, "The black community was not ready for a female minister. After six months, I knew I'd never be a pastor or have my own church. The time just wasn't right for me."

Supported by her religious credentials, Mary found part-time work supporting weddings and funerals, teaching in church-sponsored schools, supervising children at Fresh Air Fund camps, working with children at risk, and organizing and managing seasonal special events at churches. She was in great demand.

While working for the churches, Mary supported programs which cared for the elderly and the disabled. She understood the demands of providing care for persons in need. She found part-time work in clinics and care facilities. She had answered my ad for the same reason as did Emma and the others who responded: the potential for an easier job with a better environment and better pay.

My mother loved Mary and so did I. She had an exceptionally calm and peaceful personality. She radiated joy and happiness. She was loving and loyal. When my mother napped, Mary read her family Bible, full of tabbed pages, highlighter markings and penned notes in the margins. There were occasions when I would come home for lunch or some other reason and find my mother asleep and Mary reading. She concentrated so intently and was so absorbed in what she was reading that she did not notice me in the room with her.

Mary lived about 15 miles south of Clear Lake in Texas City in a home which she shared with her father, then in his mid-80's. He was healthy, drove a car, attended Masonic Lodge meetings and had no physical or mental issues. A long-time widower, Mary was his primary companion. She shopped for groceries, made most of the meals, did the laundry and maintained the home less any work which required tools. That was her father's contribution in addition to trapping and disposing of any critters that found their way into the home. Not only her father but also most of their neighbors reacted when Mary screamed at the sight of a garden snake, rat snake, tree frog or lizard which found its way into the home.

She drove a 1985 Cadillac which devoured fuel and almost always was in need of repair. On several occasions Mary would call me with car problems. I either would drive to her home to bring her to work or pick her up in a parking lot where she had left the car. There was a second vehicle at my home, and I always offered it to her to use until repairs were made on the Cadillac. She never took advantage of the offer. I asked her why she did not buy something in better condition, more fuel efficient and more economical. She told me, "Mister Pelosi, I need my Cadillac."

Frequently, on the way to work, Mary would stop at a bakery and buy muffins to share with my mother at breakfast and pastries to share with her at lunch. Mary never would accept any compensation for the food items she brought to share.

She also never accepted any compensation when she brought my mother blouses, skirts and jewelry which she purchased at a high-end second-hand store in Clear Lake on the weekends. The first time she made a purchase there, she had taken my mother with her one day during the week. She stopped doing that only because the aisles were too narrow to maneuver the wheelchair. That was also my experience the first time I brought my mother to the store. I learned why Mary shopped there. The merchandise was stylish, well-made and very affordable.

As I had done with Emma, I offered Mary the use of a credit card whenever she wanted to break up the day at home and go out for lunch. The card was kept in an envelope in the kitchen. I recommended several local restaurants most of which Mary knew. My standard for selecting a restaurant was no buffets, no fast-food places, and only those with tablecloths and silverware. No plasticware. In Clear Lake, there were more than a dozen quality restaurants.

Mary and my mother took lunch out an average of once every other week. One Saturday, I returned with my mother to one of our favorite restaurants that they had visited. The manager came to our table and told me that she was surprised to see my mother with Mary and without me once or twice in the past month or two. She added that she also was surprised to see her use my credit card for payment. But she assumed that since my mother was present everything was in order. Her final comment to me was, "Mary doesn't tip." I told her that I would work on that.

Mary told me that she didn't mind using my money for shared food and beverages for which she knew the cost, but having to calculate a tip amount with my money was something else. Her final comment on this subject with me was, "Mister Pelosi, please don't ask me to do math after I've had a good time out with your Mama."

Our neighborhood Homeowners Association provided a huge lap and small splash pool for its residents and their guests. It opened just before Memorial Day and closed just after Labor Day during the time when the older neighborhood children, trained as lifeguards, would be free from school and available to work. It was closed when I arrived in Clear Lake with my mother in September 2000.

But in Galveston, only 22 miles and 40 minutes away by car, there was the massive San Luis Resort, Spa and Conference Center, located right on the beach, which hosted a year-round heated outdoor pool. On weekends, when the weather was supportive, I would bring my mother there. Poolside were the restrooms, one of which was a family and handicapped facility. There, I would change my mother into her swimsuit. I would move her in the wheelchair to one of the access areas, lift her, and carry her into the pool supported by the safety rail which I held with one hand.

In the pool, I would stand behind her with my arms under hers and walk her back and forth in the shallow area for 30 minutes or more. Also in the pool were a series of steps on which some folks sat and sipped drinks from plastic glasses. I was able to seat my mother on those steps, move in front of her and exercise her legs and arms. From the pool, we would rest in the shade on well-padded chaise lounges using towels provided by the resort. My mother would nap, after which we would have lunch at the poolside restaurant. I changed her back into her regular clothes before we called it a day and drove home. The annual pass for access to the resort's amenities cost only $200. per family. We went as often as possible when the weather cooperated until our community pool opened on Memorial Day.

On the trip to Galveston we would drive through Texas City where Mary lived. One day we decided to surprise her and visit. She was sitting home alone reading, having just finished a variety of indoor chores. We offered to bring her to the resort to spend the afternoon with us but she declined. "Mister Pelosi. I don't have a swimsuit. I don't even own shorts. I don't do too well in the sun. And you know what? I'm afraid of the water. I can't swim."

On other occasions we would call Mary before we departed for Galveston. If she were free in the afternoon and wanted to go out to lunch with us, then we would make a date to meet her after our time at the resort. Mary knew the nice restaurants in Texas City. My mother always was hungry after the exercise routine in the pool and tired after she ate. She slept in the car on the way home and napped after we returned.

Our community pool was open during the summers. I brought my mother there in season each day on the weekends and every holiday when the weather was favorable. We would arrive as soon as the pool opened at 10 a.m., guaranteeing that I could secure two chaise lounges which I located in the shade as close as possible to the pool and diving board where my mother always enjoyed watching the children at play in the water and the teenagers trying to outdo each other at diving or what appeared to be diving. Many of their antics drew laughs from my mother.

At the pool, I repeated the San Luis Resort exercise routine with my mother. Absent an on-site restaurant for lunch, I would pack a cooler with food, beverages, fruit and energy bars. The cooler was placed between our chaise lounges poolside during the day.

Occasionally, a small child would visit with her parent. She would greet my mother and offer her a paper plate of homemade cookies or sweets. Other times, a child would bring her cut carrot sticks, slices of an apple or a pear, or a whole orange or tangerine. My mother never lost her ability to acknowledge the gesture and say, "Thank you."

On Saturdays, we would depart the pool at 2 p.m. At home, I would change my mother into her go-to-meeting clothes. She'd take a short nap for about an hour after which we would depart for the 4:30 p.m. Mass.

At St. Clare of Assisi Roman Catholic Church, there were two extra-wide pews on each side of the church which could accommodate a wheelchair. I would bring my mother to the same pew each week and transfer her to the aisle-side corner seat where I had placed a soft cushion. In 2000, when my mother first came to Mass with me, she was able greet our fellow parishioners. She also was able to stand, but never kneel, during parts of the Mass. She could sing the hymns and recite the prayers which she knew. She lost that ability slowly as the Parkinson's took a firmer grasp of her senses. But she never lost her ability to accept the Communion wafer presented to her by the priest or Eucharistic minister.

I always sat to my mother's right and helped her to stand when she was able. When seated during the sermons, I usually took out my checkbook and paid bills. I never thought that a man who had 12 more years of education beyond the university degree, worked at a respectable job, owned and maintained four homes, paid his taxes, and cared for his disabled parent needed to be told by someone half his age how to behave. I do believe that all religions are fine if they make someone feel better about themselves and act better within their society. It is what people do in daily lives, not what they believe, that is important.

In 2013, three years after my mother had died, I was training to walk across Europe in 2014 in a demonstration of support for our veterans. I walked 15 miles a day in all kinds of weather beginning and ending in my neighborhood. On good-weather days, some of the neighbors, seeing me frequently carrying a huge backpack, would stop me and ask me what I was doing. Some recognized me from the pool. They told me that they enjoyed watching us together, several adding that my mother was very lucky to be cared for in such a manner when she was in need. Usually I responded that her care was not a result of luck but of what her family sensed as obligations due to their parents in need from their children.

Mary was at the age where she still experienced hot flashes. Usually she used her bathroom to splash water on her face. Sometimes she took a quick cool shower. At times other than when we would suffer the unbearable heat and humidity of summer in Texas, she would step outside on the front walkway. There she would twist her body from side to side and wave her arms sideways and over her head. When I first saw her doing that one afternoon as I arrived home at noon, I thought that she was exercising. But I was wrong. She told me that it was her effort to try to relieve the misery which accompanies a hot flash.

At our first Christmas together, I hung the lights and arranged the decorations outdoors. I also bought a live 10-foot Norway spruce for indoors and strung lights on it. On the dining room table I left several open boxes containing tree skirts, bulbs, ornaments, tinsel, nutcrackers, holiday-themed stuffed animals, Santas, snowmen and a manger with figures. During the week, Mary and my mother could decorate the inside of the home.

Mid-morning the following Monday, Mary called me at work to tell me that she and my mother had started work on the indoor decorating. My mother told me that anything that fell on the floor, especially a stuffed Santa, reindeer or snowman, Sheba and Gizmo captured and played with as a toy.

233

Mid-week before Christmas I came home early while the women still were decorating. I took the dogs for a long walk to help keep them away from the activity inside. When we were returning home, I saw Mary standing on the front walkway twisting her torso and waving her arms in the image of her reacting to another hot flash. But I also saw her raising her legs and kicking them forward and backward. That was something new. I assumed that this must be her response to an especially severe hot flash.

As I usually do at the end of a walk when we were on our street and within 50 yards of the home, I unleashed Sheba and Gizmo. They would race down the street, up the driveway, pass through the gate and stop short at the back door.

As I got closer, Mary started shouting, "Mister Pelosi, Mister Pelosi, there's a squirrel in the house! There's a squirrel in the house! Didn't you see me signalin'? Mister Pelosi, I been standin' here signalin' since you come down the street. Didn't you see me signalin'?"

I said, "Mary, I thought you were having one of your hot flashes and a really bad one with all the jumping around you were doing. I couldn't tell that you were signaling."

Mary twisted her torso and waved her arms then said as she demonstrated, "Mister Pelosi. This is a hot flash."

Then she made the same movements again, but also picked up her legs and made the kicking movements, announcing: "Mister Pelosi. This is signalin'!"

"Mister Pelosi. There's a squirrel in the house!"

Apparently, the squirrel got into the house when Mary left the back door open to trash the Christmas wrapping paper. When she saw the squirrel inside, she left my mother seated on the sofa and ran out the back door, again leaving it open.

Sheba and Gizmo were not used to finding the back door open. When they did, they went inside. Sheba sensed and found the squirrel. When I came into the house, my mother's head was moving rapidly up, down, left, and right, and she was laughing as she watched the two dogs chase the squirrel in and out of the living room.

The squirrel ran through all the rooms, primarily the living room and dining room where there were the most windows and brightest light. It jumped on and over everything and trashed the decorations. Sheba and Gizmo stayed in very close pursuit. It jumped onto the Christmas tree; got its foot or something caught in the tree lights; and jumped down, taking the tree and a string of lights with it. The squirrel escaped from the wire, then jumped on to the fireplace mantel where tinsel, nutcrackers, stuffed animals, and other decorations fell to the floor like bombs raining down on the dogs in pursuit.

235

Mary had used her key to come in through the front door. I saw her run into the bedroom, then heard the door slam shut and the words, "Come get me when he's gone!"

I used a broom to swat at and near the squirrel hoping to guide it to one of the two open doors. After about 10 minutes of pure chaos, the squirrel ran out the front door and up the closest live oak tree. Sheba and Gizmo followed, but their prey was gone.

I gave Mary the "All Clear!" She went huffing and puffing into the back bedroom and slept for almost an hour.

My mother still was laughing when I was trying to dress down and discipline the dogs. She told me, "James, they were only trying to help you get the squirrel outside."

Before Mary departed, I asked her if she were planning to return to work tomorrow. She said, "Sure, Mister Pelosi. This is my job. Make sure them dogs stay here. They's good protection."

For a short time before dinner and an hour or so afterwards, my mother and I restored the home and the decorations. Everything was in order when Mary returned the following morning.

During the second year of her employment, Mary called me at work sounding very agitated. She was calling from the breakfast table where my mother had dropped her spoon, closed her eyes and slumped to her left side. Mary called to tell me that she had just completed an emergency 9-1-1 call. She thought that my mother was having a stroke.

I informed my coworkers then drove home covering the four-mile distance in about seven minutes. When I arrived, there were no emergency vehicles in front of the home. After I entered, Mary said, "Mister Pelosi, you done beat the ambulance here. What's the matter with them people?" She told me about my mother's experience at the breakfast table.

Mary had relocated her to the sofa and was sitting next to her petting her face and arms. My mother's eyes were closed. As I started to talk to her, the emergency crew came through the front door and took control. Mary told them what she had observed.

Within 15 minutes the paramedics and my mother were on the way to a Houston hospital. I followed in my car. I thanked Mary, told her to take time off until I needed her at the house, and paid her for a full week.

The good news was that my mother did not have a stroke. She had a urinary tract infection. The bad news was that I had been bathing my mother incorrectly. The hospital staff told me that urinary tract infections are common in elderly females who do not completely purge any soap from the vaginal area. Soap which remains there contains the bacteria which can cause an infection. Having learned that, I continued to bathe my mother in the jacuzzi tub but without any soap anywhere in the water.

I was not permitted into the Intensive Care Unit where she remained for three days. I waved to her in the mornings when she woke; drove to work when the staff began attending to her; then returned in the evenings to greet her again before I sensed that she was asleep for the night. On the fourth day, she was relocated to a room only for observation where I stayed with her the entire day. I returned in the morning of the fifth day to wait for her discharge then we drove home. The experience had drained her. She slept immediately after we arrived and most of the weekend. She drank fluids and ate about her half of what she had been consuming daily.

Mary returned on Monday. I stayed half the morning with her. She was one step ahead of me. While she was off, she had researched the subject, "urinary tract infection." One of the first things she told me was, "Mister Pelosi. No more soap or bathing gels in the jacuzzi tub. Soap is what causes them infections."

My mother perked up quickly which I attribute to her being home in familiar surroundings again with Mary, Sheba, Gizmo and me. I encouraged Mary to bring her outside to take her mid-morning and mid-afternoon rests on the chaise lounge in the sun. There she could absorb the sunshine, breathe the fresh air, and flush away and forget the smells, sights and sounds of the hospital. There never is anything pleasant about a stay in a hospital.

In early May 2004, Mary told me some unpleasant news. Her father, age 90, had suffered a stroke and was hospitalized. He was not expected to recover. Two of her sisters now were living at the family home in Texas City. Mary wanted to keep working by day when her sisters would visit their father. She was content to visit him after she finished work. Mary told me that she knew several people, very familiar with her work with my mother and with a general idea about me and the home. She would give me their contact information and, if I desired, I could arrange for a meeting and an interview. She offered a second option which was to bring the person whom she thought was best qualified, most personable and potentially most compatible for my mother to work one day. Mary and her friend Lynn would work together and, at the end of the day after I came home, we could share information and I could make a decision. I told Mary that the option for shared work was fine and that I would pay Lynn for her day's work. Mary told me that it would not be necessary; however, I insisted that it be part of the deal. Mary added that if we all meshed, then Lynn could start work after her father died. Mary would stop working with my mother and me, and help her family with the funeral arrangements and the settlement of her father's estate.

Mid-week, Mary brought her friend and neighbor, Lynn, with her to work. I met her after I arrived home. She was very happy with her day's experience and eager to replace Mary when she departed. She was every bit as polite, dignified and professional in her manner as was Mary. Most importantly, my mother liked her, and I thought that they seemed compatible. She happily accepted the job, and would start work the morning after Mary's last day.

Retired United States Air Force Senior Master Chief Davis died six days later in the early evening shortly after Mary had arrived at the hospital. She told me that she sat by his bed and took his hand. He sensed her presence, opened his eyes, looked at his first-born child, smiled and died. Mary kissed him, then alerted the nursing staff. She called her family, me, Lynn and other friends.

I took off the next morning to meet Lynn and help her and my mother with the transition. I left for work after I bathed my mother and helped Lynn dress her for the day. Lynn called me mid-afternoon to tell me that everything was fine. It was a very considerate action that lifted my spirits. When I arrived home in the afternoon, Lynn was reading to my mother outside in the sun. Sheba and Gizmo were keeping them company. After Lynn departed for the day, I spoke with my mother. She told me that she had enjoyed her first full day with Lynn. My impression was that Mary had hit a home run when she referred and helped train Lynn to replace her.

The funeral for Senior Master Chief Davis

was held on the Saturday after his death at the Hopewell Baptist Church where he had been an active member for more than 30 years. Helen, my mother and I attended the service on a beautiful late-spring day. It was scheduled to begin at 11 a.m. We arrived a half hour early, and by then the church was packed.

A squad of Masonic Knights, in their formal dress uniforms, escorted us and other mourners from the sidewalk to the entrance of the church. From there, another squad of Knights escorted us to a pew near the front of the church where Mary had reserved space for us. The church was packed with people in every pew. Dozens more were standing along the side walls. There were at least 400 folks in attendance. Helen, my mother and I were the only three who were not African-American. No one else seemed to notice. When Mary saw me moving my mother from the wheelchair to the pew, she came and hugged and kissed her, me, and Helen whom she knew from previous visits. Following Mary, the pastor came and welcomed us to his church.

The casket was at the front center of the church and draped with an American flag. To the rear, right of the casket was another American flag, the United States Air Force flag, the flag of the Masonic Knights and the flag of Hopewell Baptist Church. There was an honor guard of two Masonic Knights and two Air Force airmen, also in their dress uniforms, at the four corners of the casket. They marched away as the service started.

241

At the Sanctuary, opposite the pulpit, was a 60-member choir. The men wore dark suits, each with a white carnation boutonnière. The women wore white choral robes, each draped with a red tippet accented with a white rose.

During and after the three-plus hour service, I thought that only a Pope could have had a more spectacular funeral. The music switched between somber and lively in response to the sentiment of the pastor's preaching. The pastor spoke for more than 30 minutes about Mary's father's dedication to the church and his lifetime of service. More music and more praise by the pastor for Senior Master Chief Davis and a long sermon about service to God, country, community, each other and the less fortunate. My mother was transfixed by the splendor of the service and the glamour of the participants. When the service concluded, the family departed first. Mary and her family stopped to thank us for attending.

At home, we all felt the need for a short, mid-afternoon nap. Then we drove for an early dinner at a local restaurant where we discussed the exceptional memorial service for Mary's truly remarkable father.

The next week, Sheba, 12 years old, died from rectal cancer. Six weeks later, Gizmo, also 12, deaf, blind and depressed after her companion's death, also died. I buried them side by side in my yard in a large, private garden. There was a border of multi-colored rose bushes mixed in with butterfly weed which

242

is a nectar plant that attracts both monarch butterflies and hummingbirds. Over the graves was a cluster of Mexican petunias which bloom all year with bright blue flowers. Ronnie and Joseph Garan sent us sympathy cards which they had prepared using crayons on drawing paper writing polite expressions of sympathy and drawing pictures of Sheba and Gizmo. I kept those cards. The home was far too quiet and much less exciting without them. My life was diminished by their loss. I still miss them.

On a Thursday, three weeks after the funeral for Senior Master Chief Davis, there was a serious incident at the Space Center. The employees were sheltered in place then sent home as a safety precaution. I arrived about 2 p.m., only about an hour after I had left home to return to work following my regular noon-time chores with my mother and the dogs. Lynn asked me if I had forgotten something. I told her about the incident. Then I told her that she was free to leave for the day, something I always had done with Emma and Mary whenever I came home earlier than expected.

At 8 p.m. that evening I received a telephone call from Lynn. She told me that she was in her vehicle passing through Jacksonville, Florida, and driving north on Interstate I-95 enroute to her sister's home in South Carolina. She said that when she returned home, three hours earlier than when she was expected, she saw an unfamiliar car parked in the driveway.

After she went into her home, she heard some

noise in the bedroom and found her husband in the company of another woman. She made a beeline for the clothes closet on one side of the bed while the miscreants jumped out of the bed on the other side and fled. From the bedroom, Lynn packed as much of her clothing as would fit in her two suitcases and loaded them in the trunk of her car. With the offenders out of the house and long gone, she returned to retrieve everything of value that she wanted with her wherever she would be living next, loaded up the car, and drove away.

I asked her why she didn't come to my home where she knew there always had been one-half of the home, (two bedrooms, a den, and a full bath), available to her. She said, "Mister Pelosi. I thought about that. But I did not want to impose my problems on you and your mother. Right now, I'm too upset to even think about working, and I don't think I'm going to be any better any time soon."

I thanked her for her telephone call, for her extraordinary service, and I wished her well. I also asked her to call me again with a snail mail address to which I could send her pay. She never called.

After I hung up with Lynn, I called my boss and coworkers and told them why I needed to take off from work the next day. They all knew my situation at home. Most of them, including my boss, had met my mother. They told me, "Take as much time as you need."

I needed only one day.

The next day I called the woman whom I had ranked #3 after the five interviews. Both Emma and Mary had experience caring for strangers in rehab and health care facilities. But this woman did not. However, she had an excellent resumé on which she had written that she was "available immediately." She did have experience caring for elderly relatives and friends at their homes. At the resumé, she had attached an outstanding letter of recommendation from the pastor of the church which she and her family attended in rural Texas. Now she lived in Pasadena, just under a 30-minute commute along only three roads between her home and ours.

Mrs. Deborah Schooley is five months younger than I. She and her older sister were raised by their parents in rural Texas. As a child, she enjoyed the outdoors, the company of her family, and critters of all kinds. She was not too thrilled with public school but liked Bible school on Sundays and Bible Studies camp in the summers. She told me that "I pretty much learned all the books in the Bible." I was impressed because I knew only the first five, beginning with Genesis and ending with Deuteronomy. I asked her if she still remembered any of them and could tell me their names. She said, "Sure. The Old Testament and The New Testament." I knew then that she would be a good companion for my mother. She was better than good. She was exceptional.

Deborah came to work on Monday. As I had done with Mary and Lynn, I took off the first half of the day to help her get started. The easiest way for me to do that was to demonstrate how I performed each of the tasks.

Sharing Mary's sentiments about an automobile, she arrived driving an older model Cadillac. When I saw it pull up in front of the house, I thought that Mary had returned to visit. Much like the condition of Mary's Cadillac, Deborah's leaked oil, the reason why they both kept their cars parked curbside. The similarities extended to the early morning or evening telephone calls when Deborah would tell me that the Cadillac had broken down. I always provided her transportation for as long as she needed it, and I offered to fund the repairs which she refused. She refused, too, the offer to use my spare automobile until hers was repaired.

She brought her pet dog with her. Chaz was a charcoal-colored toy poodle, purchase price $600., discounted from $800. He was so small that he was able to walk between the bars of the wrought iron fence which enclosed the yard, and escape to roam around the new neighborhood. That night, I bought chicken wire and fastened it across the base of the fence high enough to keep Chaz confined to the yard. He was full of energy and spent most of the morning exploring the home and yard. He would rotate sitting next to Deborah or my mother on the sofa or chair in the living room. Often, when my mother slept on the sofa, he slept at her feet. All of six pounds, it was easy for my mother to hold and pet him or to move him out of her lap if he had sat or slept there too long.

Deborah was divorced from her first husband, Rick, a Navy veteran and contractor, with whom they raised three sons: Benjamin, Timothy, and David. Over time, as I heard stories about her boys, it seemed to me that she was overgenerous with her attention and support for them. She helped fund new vehicles after they wrecked theirs. She loaned them money for things such as a used motorcycle, weapons, car insurance and repairs, and past-due rent payments.

I considered their selfishness and, as grown men, their seeming dependence upon their mother for financial support as border-line abusive and juvenile. After each new story about the cookie jar being emptied, I suggested that she kick the kids from the nest and let them work to make it on their own. Deborah had no alimony from Rick, very little savings, and a wait of 15 years before she would be eligible to receive early Social Security.

She remarried not too long after the divorce. Her second husband, Billie, was an industrial mechanic. He had a daughter by his first marriage, several years older than Deborah sons. She lived on her own in another state. Billie and the boys had a difficult relationship together at home. The boys moved away when they could afford to, usually finding someone with whom to share an apartment. Benjamin enlisted in the Navy, then married. His two younger brothers remained locally in the Clear Lake area.

Deborah was every much as professional, competent, responsible, reliable, caring and loving as was Mary. The was some greater degree of compatibility between my mother and Deborah than there was with Mary only because of a more similar experience in their challenging childhood years, and their shared experience of raising three children very close in age. Mary never had married.

Also, it also was easier for my mother and Deborah to identify with the old movies which often occupied two hours of their day together. The romance stories and musicals of the 30's, 40's and 50's starred predominantly white actors and actresses. While I watched many of them with my mother, I often wondered how any person of color could enjoy, relate to, or even tolerate such babble and baloney. Given the trash that Hollywierd produces today, I, most of my family and many of my friends are unwilling or unable to tolerate the new generation of babble and baloney even with well-integrated casts acting in stories about romance with scenes that include love-making in plots that I thought were found only in magazines which came with centerfolds.

Deborah always arrived for work dressed immaculately. She wore a watch but no other jewelry which would interfere with working. When my mother napped, she would play outdoors for a short time with Chaz. She found time to clean the house, a chore that I never required of her. It embarrassed me sometimes when I returned to find the refrigerator or stove cleaned, the floors swept, the carpets vacuumed, the knick-knacks dusted and the bathrooms GI'd. I thought that I had been doing a fairly good job on my own. Apparently it was not good enough for a woman who kept house for a husband and three sons.

On occasion Deborah would leave the home by the front door to retrieve something from her vehicle. When she did so, Chaz would run out the door with her. Unlike Sheba and Gizmo, Chaz was not trained to respond to voice commands, and, if he were, he did not obey them. At noon one Thursday, while I was home for the lunch chores, Deborah went outside and Chaz followed her. At the same time that Chaz spotted a squirrel across the street in the neighbor's driveway, another neighbor, in some sort of rush, was speeding down the road. Chaz's charcoal color matched the color of the macadam road. The driver did not see him dash across the street until it was too late. From the kitchen I heard the screech of fast-braking tires. I ran out to see Deborah kneeling by Chaz's tiny crushed body and my neighbor apologizing profusely to her. I wrapped Chaz's body in a small blanket compliments of United Airlines and, while holding him, told Deborah to go home and take off the next day, Friday, from work. She took Chaz's body from me, placed him on the front passenger's seat, thanked me and drove away.

I went inside, called my office, and told

my team why I would not return to work that day or the next. Then I served lunch to my mother, did the dishes and tended to her hygiene. While she was reclining on the sofa, I sat beside her, placed her lower legs and feet on my thighs and massaged them. I told her about the accident with Chaz. She was noticeably affected. I moved from the sofa when she fell asleep.

Deborah came to work the next day, sadly blaming herself for Chaz's death but not evidently still grieving although her eyes were very red. She told me that spending the day staying busy with my mother would be the best way for her to feel better. She added, "James, your mother is my best friend now. I don't want to be anywhere else today."

I was very happy to hear that. I was not so thrilled knowing that I would be returning to work.

Deborah was the first of the care providers who addressed me as "James." Several times I had asked Emma, Mary and Lynn to do so, but none of them would. It never has been my style to stand on formality, especially in my home.

Earlier in the narrative I had written that the garden plot where I had buried Sheba and Gizmo was a mesh of rose bushes, Mexican petunia's and milkweed which, as a nectar plant, attracts monarch butterflies and hummingbirds. I often saw them when I maintained the yard and garden. I transplanted several stalks of the milkweed to pots and located the pots on the patio. I hoped that from the kitchen or outside on the patio, my mother and the aide would be able to watch the butterflies and hummingbirds.

Almost a dozen hummingbirds included my patio as part of their territory. Competitors buzzed each other at the hummingbird feeders and at the milkweed pots. Hundreds of monarch butterflies began their new lives there, transformed from caterpillars which fed on the milkweed. When ready, a nourished caterpillar will find by instinct a secure place on which to create a chrysalis, in which it will be transformed into a butterfly in about three to four weeks.

I noticed a chrysalis forming beneath the frame of a window at the kitchen. As it began to change colors from emerald green with its golden band to black, I knew that soon a butterfly would emerge. I alerted Deborah to be watchful. She told me, one day after I had arrived home at the end of work, that she and my mother had witnessed the miracle of a butterfly emerging from its chrysalis.

I asked her what they had seen. She told me, "Well, we saw the black-shaped thing (chrysalis) start to wiggle. We moved up real close to the window to watch. Then the horns came out. (I knew she meant "antennae.") In a little bit out came its paws ("legs") and nose ("proboscis") and then its body and wings. But it didn't fly away. It looked like it fell down, so we went outside. We found it on the ground fanning its wings. Then it flew up to the fence, fanned its wings some more and flew up and away over the garage. I've never seen anything like that before."

I returned home for lunch one glorious spring afternoon, expecting to find Deborah and my mother sitting outside in the sun. But they were inside, sitting together on the sofa. Deborah was rubbing my mother's stomach. I asked if anything were wrong. Deborah told me that my mother seemed somewhat slow in her movements during the morning and, although she had eaten her full breakfast, she complained of a stomach ache. Having heard that, I called the family doctor and was able to secure his last appointment for the day.

Deborah and I drove together with my mother to the doctor's office. His nurse took her vital signs. Her weight, blood pressure and heart rate were normal, but she had a slightly elevated temperature. Deborah described her observations of my mother during the day. The doctor suspected a gall bladder issue, in part because my mother's pain center was exactly in the area where the gall bladder is located. He told us to drive to the local hospital, only eight miles from his office, and go the Emergency Room which we did.

The Emergency Room team was expecting us. While I provided the administrators my mother's personal information, Deborah stayed with her. From the Emergency Room, she was admitted and provided a private room. After she was settled, Deborah drove home and I stayed. I called my sisters in Florida and informed them of her status. I also called Deborah to tell her that she was not needed until sometime after my mother returned home.

The operation to remove the gall bladder was performed the following morning. There were no issues. A nurse told me that my mother's vital signs were strong throughout the operation. After the operation, she was moved to the Intensive Care Unit for observation and, after six hours, returned to her room. She remained there only one more day and then was discharged.

At home, my mother made a quick recovery, regaining her appetite and settling into her routine. I gave all the credit to Deborah for her loving care and attention.

Deborah took her summer vacation when I was required to travel to Europe for work. Then my sisters either would travel from Florida to care for our mother or I would bring her to them. In the years when my sisters came to Clear Lake for the summer, I would bring my mother to Florida for two weeks at Christmas when Deborah would have an additional two-week vacation.

There was one occasion when I was required to make a one-week trip to Europe on no notice. My sisters were not available to support me, but Deborah told me that she would be willing to do double duty. For one week, she cared for my mother around the clock. I doubled her salary and gave her my check book and credit card. I told her to contact an agency, such as Visiting Angels, if she needed time off or if the strain were too difficult. She did so only once during that week.

After I returned, Deborah told me that she had needed someone to watch my mother for two or three hours while she resolved a medical problem related to her mother. She called Visiting Angels and was shocked at the hourly wage, approximately three to four times what the care provider received from that employer. Apparently, most of the exorbitant fee went for advertising, insurance, infrastructure and overhead. Deborah told me that when she came back to the home, "I saw the woman asleep in the chair and your mother asleep on the sofa. The television was on. You mother woke up when I came in, but the woman from Visiting Angels did not. I woke her and told her to leave. I refused to pay her and told her to have the agency call you after you returned." No one from Visiting Angels called me, and I never again called that agency.

Deborah knew that every Saturday afternoon I would bring my mother to the 4:30 p.m. Mass at St. Clare of Assisi Roman Catholic Church only a two-mile, five-minute drive from our home. On this recent trip to Europe, when Deborah was caring for my mother, she took her to Mass.

The parish priest once asked me if my mother would like to attend Confession. I said, "I don't think she ever has done anything in her life that was sinful and needs confessing."

Then Father Dominic asked, "How about you?"

I told him that I was guilty of the same sin every week: "Thinking impure thoughts."

Deborah also knew that every Wednesday I had a 5:30 p.m. appointment with Tammy at the beauty salon where my mother would have her hair washed and set. She brought her there for her appointment during the week that I was away in Europe. Deborah was so impressed with Tammy that she dropped her beautician in favor of her.

There was one week when the salon was closed as the result of flooding caused by a burst water pipe. Having watched and supported the routine performed by Tammy, I thought that I could do the same work. Everything I needed was at our home. My sisters had left two sets of curlers and a blow dryer from their visits.

I draped two towels over my mother, then washed and rinsed her hair. I remembered how Tammy would part her hair in sections and roll her hair onto the curlers. I tried that with one section at the front, two sections at each side, and two sections (top and bottom) at the back. Then I relocated my mother to the living room; turned on a tape of a Fred Astaire and Ginger Rogers musical, and let my mother watch the show while I blow dried her hair. The movie was 90 minutes. I felt my mother's hair after an hour. It was dry and so I stopped.

Back in the bathroom, I unfastened each of

the curlers while my mother watched in the mirror. When I finished, something didn't look right. It appeared as if no two rolls of dry hair were the same size and shape. They looked like a mass of hairy mangled corkscrews. I hoped that everything would look better after I combed, brushed and teased her hair as I had seen Tammy do. The result was something which looked like a mix between the hair styles of Buckwheat from *The Little Rascals* and Curly from *The Three Stooges*.

My mother leaned forward in the wheelchair to get a closer look at what I had done. Watching her look into the mirror, turn her head to each side, pause and look again, then touch her hair with each hand, I started to feel somewhat better at the result. That is, until she started laughing. The more I apologized, the more she laughed. Somehow Deborah was able to undo the damage the next morning. That was the last time I ever tried to care for my mother's hair.

When I returned from Europe, Deborah had a new pet. Jet was identical in size and color to Chaz and just as manic. When I saw him, I asked Deborah to keep him leashed whenever he went outside anywhere other than the enclosed yard. She told me, "I'm one step ahead of you on that. I had to go to three different pet shops to find a collar small enough to fit him."

The first Sunday in February 2007 was Super Bowl Sunday. The morning started out to be a spectacular day weather-wise: bright sunshine and cool, maybe 50 degrees F. After breakfast and hygiene, I dressed my mother in a camisole, long-sleeve blouse, light button-down sweater and slacks. I brought her outside on to the patio and moved her from the wheelchair to the chaise lounge with her face in the shade and the rest of her body in the sun.

There were two vehicles parked in our garage: a new Saturn Vue SUV and a 40-year old classic Mercedes Benz 450 SL coupe. I backed the Saturn down the driveway about 20 yards from the garage and the Mercedes about 10 yards away. Then I moved everything else out from the garage and started to clean it.

I decided to take a short break, and went inside to get something to drink for my mother and me. We sat together for a while. I told her what I was doing in the garage and how the work was long overdue. When I came from the patio to the driveway I saw two boys, in their late teens or early 20's, standing between the two vehicles. I never had seen them before in the neighborhood. I asked if I could help them. They answered, "No, just looking." Then I asked them if they were planning to watch the game today. They turned and walked down the driveway without answering me.

Not more than 15 minutes later, while I was working in and out of the garage, they passed again, stopped and looked up the driveway. As I headed towards them, they turned around and walked away.

Later, while I was standing on the ladder which leads into the attic inside the garage, I heard the sounds of something impacting. To me, it sounded as if mortar rounds were exploding quite some distance away. I climbed down the ladder and was shocked at what I saw.

From the yard behind our home, large, heavy logs were sailing over the garage and impacting on the driveway, some only a yard or two from the Mercedes, but others only a few feet from my mother. There were three logs on the patio within a yard of the chaise lounge. My mother had been peppered with wooden shards, and she was holding her arms crossed at her chest and her hands over her face. There were wooded shards on the pavement surrounding her, others on her body and two or three protruding from the left sleeve of her sweater. I took the sweater off her and saw blood stains on the sleeve of her blouse.

I looked closely at the rest of my mother's body and there did not appear to be any other injuries. Then I ran to the eight-foot wooden fence at the back of my yard, jumped and held myself at the top, and saw the same two boys who had been on my property about to hurl more logs. I yelled, "I'm coming to get you and I'm packing." (The "packing" part was not true.)

I ran past my mother and around the corner, dialing 9-1-1 on my cell phone as I ran. In front of the home from which the logs were being hurled, I saw two cars I did not recognize. I gave the 9-1-1 dispatch operator the makes, models, and license plate numbers. The boys ran out the front door and dashed to those two vehicles. I yelled at them, "You tried to kill my mother. I'll get you both."

Within five minutes, while I was treating the bleeding at my mother's face and arms, two Harris County Deputy Sheriff vehicles arrived at my home. The officers found me in the yard. While I described the incident, I showed them my mother's wounds at the left side of her face, her left-side forearm and upper arm. We agreed that she did not need immediate medical attention; however, an ambulance did arrive, having been summoned by the 9-1-1 dispatcher. The paramedics cleaned and bandaged my mother's injuries.

While one officer sped away to pursue the assailants, the other stayed with me. He recorded my description of the events; and, photographed my mother's injuries, the logs and wood shards on the pavement, and the pile of logs in the neighbor's yard. While he was taking the photographs, I scaled the fence and threw four logs over it into the back of my yard. I wanted to be able to identify in court that the logs hurled between the properties that injured my mother were from the same source.

In the evening, I called Deborah and told her the events of the day. She came over and visited with us helping to ease my mother's distress and promising always to protect her.

The offenders were caught. They, and the teenage girl who had been alone at home with them that Sunday morning while her divorced mother was away for the day, all told different stories when questioned by the police. The boys were tried separately on multiple charges. I brought my mother to court each time that I testified against them. No one expected her to testify.

They were convicted and jailed. I received a nice settlement for my mother's injuries from the neighbor's insurance company which provided coverage, mandatory because the family had a mortgage on their property.

Later that month, Deborah's husband was diagnosed with cancer. He worked a reduced schedule and was home two or three days during the week. Occasionally Deborah would leave to visit him at their home in Pasadena when I was back from work to bathe and feed lunch to my mother. In late-spring, Billy was admitted to the hospital. He went in and out of the hospital for chemo treatments for almost three months. One Saturday during the summer, I drove my mother to visit him and Deborah at the hospital. He died in mid-July.

Deborah was devasted, not at the loss of her husband, but at his treachery in the months before his death. When he first was diagnosed in January, he had all the bills associated with operating their home, including the mortgage, sent to his place of business instead of the family home. Then he stopped paying everything except the utilities. He changed his will and left the home, which

Deborah expected to inherit, to his daughter from his first marriage. Deborah did not discover any of this until one day in August, about three weeks after his death, when one of his friends from work brought her all the mail containing the unpaid bills, including a notice of pending foreclosure on the property. Only a day or two after that shock, Billy's daughter called her and told her to vacate the property. She was enroute to sell it.

I did not want to lose Deborah. My first reaction was to offer her the opportunity to live with my mother and me. She said that she did not want to do that primarily because it would be difficult whenever her sons would come to visit. She thought it best if each of us had a little time away from one another. Next, I offered to help her find an apartment locally and offered to pay the rent. That, too, she rejected saying that it was too generous and she could not reconcile the difference between the evil deeds done to her by her husband with the generosity offered by her employer.

But I lost her. Deborah decided that she would return to her childhood home near Waco, Texas and live with her mother. "Mama's going to need some help soon."

Mother Earlene was 85, maintained the home and garden, drove to Walmart where she worked as the outdoor attendant at the fuel station, climbed ladders to wash the windows and fix the roof, and chased away potentially rabid feral animals with a broom.

I asked Deborah if she would stay long enough for me to find a replacement and, of course, she agreed.

Recovering the interview notebook, now for the fourth time, I called the woman whom I ranked #4. I was surprised that, after six years, she answered the telephone and remembered me. I was even more surprised when she told me that she was available. Sharon had a solid resumé which included duty as a guard at the Texas State prison in Huntsville, care for her parents, work as an aide at nursing homes and rehabilitation centers and clerical work in a clinic. She was divorced with no children at home. She had a son in junior college near Dallas. She said that she was available immediately, adding that she did not have to give any prior notice to her current employer.

I asked her to come to the home where she had interviewed at 8 a.m. on Monday. I gave her the address and directions. Now I had three days to help my mother and Deborah ease their separation after more than three years together as good friends.

Once more, I stayed home from work to orient and help Sharon. At first, my mother was slightly distant from her, probably missing Deborah and Jet and also as a result of the tighter hold which the Parkinson's disease was having on her now after seven years. But Sharon was energetic and full of life. She was shorter than Deborah but in the same physical proportions. She had an athlete's physique with strong arms and legs. She could maneuver my mother as easily as could Mary and Deborah.

After two weeks, Deborah called me to tell me that she was back in Clear Lake. She and her mother had not been managing well together. She told me, "Mother is just too set in her ways for me. I needed to leave."

She packed and moved to Seabrook, only about four miles from our home. She was living with her middle son, Timmy, who was training to become a Deputy Sheriff. During the day, she was looking for an affordable apartment. I asked her if she wanted to return, and she told me, "No. You have someone else now and I'm still not settled with everything."

Just over three weeks had passed and the Labor Day weekend was approaching. Sharon's son had finished his studies and had enlisted in the Air Force. On the day after Labor Day, he would ship out to his first basic training duty station. On the Monday before Labor Day, Sharon asked me if she could have off on the Tuesday following the holiday. She said that when she finished work on Friday, she would start the drive north to Dallas. She wanted "to be with my baby" for the Labor Day weekend and then say her "Farewell" when he left for training the next morning. She would drive back to Clear Lake on Tuesday after his departure, and be back at work on Wednesday. I said that would be fine.

I was seated at the kitchen table feeding my mother dinner when Sharon returned after work Friday at about 7 p.m. She knocked on the back door and came inside. She said, "Mister Pelosi. I just want to wish you both a happy Labor Day weekend, and give your mother a hug before I leave. I'll miss her." She moved to my mother and hugged her.

I stood up, shook her hand and told her to have a safe trip and a good time with her son of whom she should be very proud. "The Air Force has great training, great opportunities, and great traditions. I hope he stays and makes a career with the military."

She said, "Thank you." Then she pulled a pistol from her purse, pointed it at me and said, "Mister Pelosi, I have to ask a favor. May I have some money, please?" Very polite.

Looking at the pistol I asked her, "How much do you need?"

"Whatever you can spare."

Forty years earlier, when I was a teenager and still living at home on Long Island, my father knew that my friends and I would travel occasionally into the city to watch sporting events. Some of the neighborhoods were not so nice, especially when it got dark. He told me to carry my real wallet in my front pocket, with as little in it of value as was necessary. Then he told me to carry a "dummy wallet" with a copy of my driver's license, library card, school photo ID and a "New York roll" (a $10.00 bill wrapped around five ones and some sheets of tissue paper) in my back pocket. If ever I were robbed, I was to give up the dummy wallet, not my life.

Since that day, I always have kept a dummy wallet. I walked to the desk, removed it and gave it to her. She said, "Thank you," and put the pistol down on the table. Then she walked over to my mother, hugged her a second time and gave her a kiss. She walked past me, waved to both of us, opened the door and left, forgetting her pistol.

I left the pistol on the table.

After we finished dinner, we did the dishes together and then went to the bathroom to tend to her hygiene as was our routine. About 9:15 p.m., we were in the living room watching one of the old movies when we heard a knock on the back door.

Sharon had returned. She came in and announced, "Mister Pelosi, I forgot my pistol." I told her it still was on the table where she had left it. She said, "Thank you. See you on Wednesday," and left.

Sharon would not see us on Wednesday. About 2 a.m., well after my mother and I had gone to bed and were asleep, the landline next to my bed rang. Lieutenant Barney Fife, (I was somewhat groggy and am not exactly sure about the name), from the Walker County Sheriff's Department called. He asked, "Is this Mister James Joseph Pelosi?" I said, "Yes."

He said, "We have a Miss Sharon Gadson in custody up here in Huntsville. She had in her possession at the time of her arrest a wallet which contains a photocopy of your Florida driver's license, an expired Harris County library card, a hotel receipt from Germany, a ticket stub from a Christmas concert in Houston in 2002, and 15 dollars in cash. Are you missing that wallet?"

I said, "No. I gave it to her."

Lieutenant Fife asked me, "Why did you give it to her?"

I told him that she was pointing a pistol at me at the time that she asked me for money, and I thought it would be prudent to give her the wallet and its contents. The money was in that wallet. Everything else is expired and has no value. I don't care about the 15 dollars.

Then he asked me where this all happened. I told him, "In my home. She works for me, maybe 'worked' is the better word, helping me to care for my mother who is disabled by Parkinson's disease."

"About what time did she leave your home with the pistol and your wallet?"

I asked him, "The first time, or the second time?

"What do you mean?"

I told him, that the first time she left, it was while we were having dinner about 6:45 p.m. But she had forgotten her pistol and came back a little after 9:15 p.m. or so, while my mother and I were watching television. She remembered that she had forgotten the pistol, and came back to get it."

"And you gave it to her?"

"No, I did not. I told her that it still was on the kitchen table where she left it."

"Why didn't you keep it?

"Keep it? It wasn't mine. During my time in the military, I served in five locations where folks were shooting at me and my soldiers. I don't want to see another weapon the rest of my life, except maybe in a museum."

Lieutenant Fife told me, "We don't have any record of a 9-1-1 call or any law enforcement incident report from anywhere in Texas."

He asked, "Did you call the police?"

I answered, "I should call the police? I should help you put one more black person, obviously with some serious headspace and timing problems, behind bars and keep her there at taxpayer expense? You law enforcement people just took 10 years off the 24-year prison sentence for that bum Jeffrey Schilling who, with his Enron comrades-in-crime, stole 11 billion dollars from their investors and shareholders. That's billion with a capital B. Eleven billion dollars compared to 15 dollars. You think this is something which merits the taxpayer's attention. I don't."

He hung up on me.

Sharon, enroute to Dallas, stopped at the Huntsville prison. She timed her trip to coincide with the shift change for the guards. Apparently she intended to make some trouble for the guards whom she felt were responsible for her losing her job there. There was far more firepower among the departing guards than there was with what Sharon was packing. I don't even know if the pistol was loaded. There was no violence. No one was injured.

Sharon wrote me almost every other week from prison. In her letters she first would ask about my mother, then she would comment on the reasons why I would make a good husband, and propose marriage to me. I never answered any of those letters. I do hope that her prison sentence paled in comparison to the only 14 years for Jeffrey Schilling.

If ever I needed Deborah it was then. I knew that my mother's functionality and alertness were declining, slowly but surely. In the fall of 2007, she already had outlived her life expectancy by 10 years and her sister by six years. Aunt Kate's life had been compromised by Parkinson's disease and similar debilities. I believed that my mother still was strong, and I was hoping for another five to 10 years together with her.

I called Deborah. I told her what had happened with Sharon and said that I was desperate. I was absolutely honest when I told her that my mother may have between five and 10 years of life left, and I wanted it to be as happy and as comfortable and as full of love as possible. We still were friends. I needed her back. She said she would return to work. She surprised both of us when she visited with Jet on the weekend.

I retold the story about Sharon which she thought was remarkable, especially having heard dozens of similar such stories from her son, the Deputy Sheriff, with whom she was living. In many of those stories the outcome had ended very differently.

My finances were strong. I told Deborah that I would do whatever she wanted if the result was that she would stay with my mother and me. Earlier, when she called from her son's apartment in Seabrook to ask about my mother, she told me that she was looking for an apartment but that they were too expensive. After Billy died, I had offered to pay the rent for an apartment for her if only she would stay. Now I offered to pay the rent, any association fees, all the utilities, and her transportation costs such as the fuel and repairs to the Cadillac. Still she said, "No. Thank you. You pay me more than enough. I can make it on my own."

I told her that we three were a team and in this for the long haul. I offered to buy her a house. I suggested a two-bedroom, two-bathroom home in Clear Lake close to my home with a garage for her Cadillac and a fenced-in yard for Jet. She could host her mother or anyone else in the second bedroom. She also could care for my mother in her home on days when she wanted a change of pace or had something there to keep her busy.

I reminded her that Billy and his daughter stole her rightful home from her. I added that, if she accepted the offer, I would pay the all the costs for insurance, taxes and any and all repairs for anything. She would pay only the utilities from her salary.

The next weekend, after she had returned to work, assuming the routine as if she never had been gone, we three drove through Clear Lake looking at the different neighborhoods.

For one day on each of the next three weekends, we kept looking. Deborah found a nice, one story, 1500 square foot home with two bedrooms and two bathrooms, (one bedroom and bathroom on each side of the home), a large eat-in kitchen, and adjoining living room and dining room. The property included a two-car garage and a fenced-in yard. It was one of four homes in a cul-de-sac which backed up to a green belt where Jet could play and a community lap pool where he could not.

I made an offer very close to the asking price with a fair sum of money to be deposited as good faith in escrow. On the contract, I declared that I would pay the balance of the purchase price in cash at the closing given favorable results, that is, no issues with the home inspection report and the pest report, both of which I paid to have done.

Both reports came back without issue. We set

a date and time for closing, early afternoon on a Friday. I planned to come home for lunch as usual, then take the remainder of the work day off to support the closing and a post-closing celebration dinner. At lunch I was all excited. Deborah seemed a bit down. I thought that perhaps she was tired at the end of another full work week.

In the bathroom, while I was in the tub bathing my mother, Deborah moved the vanity stool alongside the tub, sat down, began to cry, and said, "James, I'm sorry. I cannot do this. I cannot take the house."

While I finished bathing my mother, I tried to convince her that she deserved the home, and that my maintaining it while she lived there would not be a burden to me. I suggested delaying the closing to give her more time to think things through again, and understand everything that was involved for all of us. But as she continued to cry, I noticed that my mother was becoming increasingly upset.

I ended the discussion with the comment, "Okay, Deborah. I understand. I never want to put any pressure on you for anything. Never. I'll go to the closing alone. Everything will be fine."

Then I asked her if this decision meant that she also was giving up her job. She answered immediately, "Oh no. I love it here. I love your mother. She's no work at all. I just can't take a house from you."

At the closing, the staff was surprised. A

senior closing agent with over 30 years' experience said, "It's the same as the 'runaway bride' syndrome. A woman becomes engaged; she and her beau set the date for the wedding; they rent the hall; hire a caterer; send out the invitations; select the wedding party members; conduct the rehearsal; and attend the rehearsal dinner. The bride-to-be is a no-show at church on her wedding day."

I lost the good faith money, the expenses for the home inspection reports, and the seller sued me. But I knew that the good faith money was my defense against a lawsuit. However, I still paid my attorney to remind the seller that he had no standing. The escrow company waived its processing fees, telling me that, under the circumstances, "It's our little gift to you. Good luck. Maybe we'll meet again."

The event never again was discussed in my home. Deborah continued to rent an apartment. She would not accept any support for anything from me. She remained with us and worked without skipping a beat.

There are only four fun holidays for me when I overeat hamburgers and hot dogs and drink cold beer in moderation. They are Memorial Day, The Fourth of July, Labor Day, and Veterans' Day. As a veteran, except for Labor Day, the other three holidays have special meaning to me and most veterans.

In November 2007, the 232nd birthday of the

United States Marine Corps was Saturday the 10th; Veterans' Day was the next day, Sunday the 11th; and Veterans' Day celebrated as a U.S. Federal holiday was Monday the 12th. Deborah and I had a three-day weekend.

On Monday, November 12, our day began as usual. I had my mother up, washed, refreshed and dressed for breakfast by 8 a.m. As we were headed from the bedroom through the living room to the kitchen, the doorbell at the front door rang. We detoured and I opened the door.

Standing in front of my mother and me was a very presentable young man in his early 20's, close-cropped hair, clean shaven, dressed in military desert-sand combat boots, desert camouflage trousers and an olive drab (OD) T-shirt. I thought that he might be a veteran.

He told me that his name was Nathan. He asked me if I needed the two live oak trees at the front of my home trimmed. They stood centered, one each on the two halves of my property. I asked him, given his appearance, if he were a veteran. He told me, "No, Sir. I tried, but I could not pass the physical."

Then I said to him, "Let me show you something, Nathan." I moved with my mother out the door and stopped on the walkway.

I told Nathan that my home faces to the south and gets the sun. I showed him the large windows at four locations: master bedroom, library, front door and dining room. I showed him the front garden filled with color from annuals such as geraniums, lantanas, pentas,

273

petunias and zinnias. Then I told him that I needed the two oak trees full and thick for three reasons: they keep the house protected from the summer sun and my utility bills lower; they provide shade for the blooming colored plants and grass; and, they provide concealment from anyone looking into the windows from the sidewalk or the street.

He said that he understood. Then he told me that his wife, who was sitting in the passenger seat of his beat-up pick-up truck, was pregnant, and he needed to "make extra money for the baby."

He pointed up at some small branches and asked, "Well, Sir, what if I just trimmed out things like these and some other dead branches? Fifty dollars a tree."

He looked and sounded like any one of my young soldiers when I was in the Army. Almost all of them never had enough money, especially if they were married with children. I said, "Okay. But you see this woman here? We were just on our way to have breakfast when you rang the doorbell. She is disabled by Parkinson's disease. I need to feed her, then tend to her hygiene and give her a bath. Then I have to dress her and get her ready for the day. It may be almost two hours before I am able to get back to you. Is that Okay? Do you have to be anywhere?"

Nathan said, "No, that's fine, Sir. If I finish early, I'll find some other work close by and meet you later."

I brought my mother to the table for breakfast and we started the day. From the kitchen table, we could hear the sound of a chainsaw in operation. After breakfast, I accomplished everything that I had told Nathan would be my routine for the morning. We no longer heard the sound of a chainsaw. It was close to 10 a.m. and the end of the two-hour window when I had told Nathan that thought I would meet him.

I opened the front door and brought my mother outside. What I saw shocked me. All of the biggest base limbs, perhaps three feet in circumference, four on each tree at what once were the 12, 3, 6, and 9 positions that kept such massive trees in balance, were gone. At the next level up, all four slightly smaller limbs, perhaps two feet in circumference at the 2, 5, 8, and 11 positions were gone. The entire front of the home, extending across all the front windows and over the windows by about three feet, was exposed. From the walkway and street, I could see through the dining room deep into the kitchen, and from the library deep into the living room. Also exposed were all of the seasonal colored flowers and a good portion of the grass which, prior to the butchering, had been shaded.

Nathan's vehicle was parked across the street at a home diagonally across from mine. Nathan came down from a ladder and started to walk across the street carrying the chainsaw in his right hand. As he walked toward me, I stopped and shouted, "Nathan, did you listen to even one thing I said to you? What the hell were. . ."

At the sound of the word "hell" Nathan fired up the chainsaw and yelled as he came toward me, "I'll cut your fu**in' head off!"

Now I was at a critical impasse. I could not get back to my mother and get her into the safety of the home before he would be on me. So, recalling my training in the Army that "the best defense is a good offense," and the combatives that I had been taught at infantry and Ranger training, I rushed him and kicked him with all my power between his legs, impacting directly into that part of his body that some men I know think is more important to them than the brain.

Nathan fell in the road, grabbing at his crotch and yelling loudly enough to drown out the sound of the chainsaw bouncing in circles close to him where he had dropped it. This bought me just enough time to rush to my mother, wheel her around, get her inside and lock the door.

Nathan was at the door seconds later after I had locked it and while I was dialing 9-1-1. The dispatch operator could hear the sound of the chainsaw as Nathan cut into the front door which suffered the death of a thousand cuts. I was able to give the operator his name, physical description and a description of his pick-up truck. Then Nathan moved from the door, retrieved his ladder and started to cut down all the tree limbs which he could reach on both trees.

His final act as a madman was to girdle each of the two trees. Girdling is the process of cutting around a tree about three feet up from the ground and making the cut deep enough to kill the tree's ability to move water and nutrients through its roots up into the tree. It's like severing arteries for a tree but, instead of an immediate death, it is a slow, painful process choking the lifeline of a tree. Nathan fled after this additional act of cruelty.

After the log incident a few years earlier, two Harris County Deputy Sheriff vehicles responded. Now, five vehicles responded. Two surveyed the property, which looked like a cross between the woods outside of Foy after the German bombardment during the Battle of the Bulge and the aftermath of a Category 4 hurricane, then drove away.

A Deputy from one vehicle examined my mother. A Deputy from a second vehicle took my statement. A Deputy from the third vehicle asked the ever-increasing number of neighbors assembled in front of our home if they had seen anything related to the incident. He took some statements.

When my neighbors gathered to survey the damage and learn the cause, all the men asked me why, after I had returned my mother to safety in the home, I did not grab a weapon and shoot Nathan while he was destroying my property. I told them, "I don't own any weapons."

After I said that, the collective response was, "What? Are you crazy?" This is Texas."

One by one, six of my neighbors went back to their homes, all located on my street, and returned with firearms. They were displayed on the undisturbed area of my front lawn and the driveway. The six men got into a discussion about which sort of weapon would have been most appropriate for this incident.

The retired Air Force Major suggested a 45-caliber pistol for its firepower. "One shot anywhere to the body and he's down!"

The banker urged using a Glock pistol. "It's lightweight and rapid fire. Expend every round in the chamber and he's gone."

The former refugee from Vietnam, who worked with me at NASA, recommended a shotgun. "Yeow havva showgun en yeow no mees. Yeow no havva no howah shoot."

Other neighbors passed by looking at the destruction, asking what had happened and adding to the debate with my other neighbors about weapons. One bystander told me, "Jim, except for the mess of tree limbs on your front lawn, I would have thought that the NRA was having a yard sale here."

At the end of the holiday, I gave my mother a second refreshing bath and we ended the day watching the musical, *"Hello Dolly."* She seemed absolutely unphased by the events of the day.

Nathan and his girlfriend (not his wife and not pregnant) were caught within four hours. Both were drug-tested and the results were positive for multiple drugs. Nathan was charged with "Communicating a terrorist threat" (I'll cut your fu**in' head off); "Felony destruction of private property" (each live oak tree was valued at $4,500.); "Malicious vandalism" (the destruction of the front door); and "Possession of controlled substances." He had been on parole for a previous offense of "breaking and entering."

At his trial, Nathan was found guilty on all four charges. As a repeat offender and parole violator, his sentence was 30 to 45 years in prison. Aside from the fact that the event occurred in a no-nonsense state such as Texas, the strongest factor which mitigated in favor of such a severe sentence was the threat that he had posed to my disabled mother.

Next year, in the fall of 2008, it was Hurricane Ike which attacked us. As with most hurricanes, it formed in the Caribbean and massed as a Category 4 storm just after Labor Day on Thursday, September 4th.

On Monday, September 8th, Ike struck Cuba. Although only 20 people were killed, the sugar cane crop was devastated; more than 40,000 homes were destroyed totally; and, another 300,000 homes were seriously damaged. Ike was the most destructive hurricane in Cuban history, causing damages estimated at over seven billion dollars.

Ike then headed into the Gulf of Mexico with Texas, Houston, my mother and me directly in its path.

"Ike is a huge storm," Texas Governor Rick Perry said. "I cannot overemphasize the danger that is facing us. It is going to do some substantial damage. It will knock out power. It will cause massive flooding."

On Wednesday, September 10th, NASA closed the Johnson Space Center, relocating Mission Control and its aircraft at Ellington Field away from the Clear Lake area. We employees were sent home, told to secure our property, and evacuate if possible.

I arrived home immediately after the evacuation order and told Deborah what I knew about the hurricane from the NASA briefings. I suggested that she secure her property and evacuate as soon as possible. She said that she planned to do so and would relocate to the safety of her mother's home, more than 100 miles northwest of Houston near Austin. Ike was expected to hit landfall in Galveston on Saturday, September 13th, which it did.

The remainder of Wednesday and all day Thursday, my mother and I prepared to evacuate. I called my sisters in Florida and told them our plans. They spoke with our mother. Thursday evening the SUV was packed.

At the console between the front seats, I packed energy bars and hard candy. In the back seat, there was one cooler packed with ice and containing perishable food, such as sandwiches and yogurt, a second cooler also packed with ice containing fruit drinks and water, a third cooler with all the supplies I anticipated using when attending to my mother's hygiene, and a fourth empty cooler to be used for all our trash. In the rear of the SUV were our two suitcases, the wheelchair, the portable toilet, and 20 half-gallon jugs of water which I anticipated using to support my mother's hygiene during our evacuation.

At first light Friday the 12th, about 6 a.m., after breakfast, hygiene and dressing, we departed. The evacuation was a logistical nightmare.

Our Plan A was to drive the 45 miles to the International Airport Houston (IAH) and fly out to any location not in the path of the hurricane. Long ago I learned in the Army that, "the only thing that won't happen is Plan A." That proved the case with us.

The usual 60-to-75-minute drive to the airport took four hours as we averaged around only 10 miles an hour. I looked at the congestion at the airport, gave up on Plan A, and drove past it on to the expansive Interstate 45 (I-45), a north-south highway which I knew connected Galveston with Dallas. My mother's first cousin, Jackie Howk, with whom, as children, she and her sister Kate spent occasional weekends at her Long Island

Home with their Uncle Willie, lived about 15 miles east of Dallas in Mesquite, Texas.

On the road, my sisters would call us with updates about the status of the storm and, more importantly, with traffic reports describing the evacuation from Houston. Except for their expressions of support, nothing they told us about the evacuation was encouraging.

Jackie did not know that we were coming. I called Helen in Melbourne. I asked her to call Jackie, alert her that we were evacuating, and ask her if there were the opportunity for us to stay with her. Helen made the contact and was very happy to tell us that Jackie would host us. I asked Helen to call her again, describe the chaos on the roadways, and tell her that we had no idea when we would arrive. Jackie was not concerned about our arrival time, only that we would arrive safely.

As we drove north, frequently stopping and averaging only between 5 and 15 miles per hour when moving, I thought, "How did anyone ever think that this country could survive a nuclear war? We were absolutely unable to evacuate only one major city, certainly a target with its huge oil refineries and distribution centers, days ahead of a threat. Everyone on this one road would be dust."

But worse, was the fact that this was 2008, 11 years after the former Soviet Union broke apart in 1989. The Berlin Wall had fallen on November 9, 1989. The Cold War had ended. The

American military had thousands of water
trucks, fuel tankers, ambulances and transport
trucks available since then, having been
decommissioned when the Soviet-Warsaw pact
threat to NATO evaporated and the NATO bases
closed.

Why were there cars stranded on both sides
of the road because service stations had run
out of gasoline? Why were there no pre-
positioned fuel trucks? Why were there no pre-
positioned water trucks along the evacuation
route? Why were there no pre-positioned
ambulances staffed by local fire department
paramedics? And, most in demand, why were
there no pre-positioned portable toilets? My
mother and I watched men, women and children
leave their cars and walk into the woods when
nature called and they needed to respond. Many
folks, mostly men, never made it into the
woods. Governor Perry's Emergency Management
Team deserved an "F," better yet an "F minus,"
for its work (?) during Hurricane Ike.

But we were prepared to fight and win. At
the start of the evacuation, about every three
or four hours, I would stop alongside the
road. I would retrieve our portable toilet and
open both the passenger door and the door
behind it which blocked the ability of anyone
to see while I tended to my mother.

I positioned the portable toilet near the
passenger seat and transferred my mother to
it. When she had finished, I used toilet paper
and fresh washcloths to clean her. Then I
dressed her with a fresh adult sanitary pad,

undergarments and slacks. When this was finished, I transferred my mother back to the passenger seat, cleaned the portable toilet, attended to the refuse, and took a break for a drink and power bar. Merging back into traffic was easy. It wasn't as if, by letting me merge, I would be slowing down some driver who needed to get someplace fast. Nothing was moving.

After another three hours, while driving north at a snail's pace, I saw a huge, blue and white "H" sign, indicating a hospital at the next exit. I drove off the highway and brought my mother into the hospital. There we had a handicapped-person's restroom to use in totally sanitary conditions away from all of the chaos of the evacuation.

About mid-way to Dallas-Mesquite, I saw a fire station and emergency vehicles ahead at another exit. We went there. The team at the station let me bring my mother into the women's restroom. When we exited, two women were standing by the door waiting for us. They told us that they had just cooked a Friday night spaghetti dinner for the crew. They invited us to join them for pasta, salad and ice cream. Even though the dinner would have been far tastier than the cold sandwiches on which we had been snacking, I declined because I knew that Jackie, then age 80, was waiting for us. But I could not say "No" to ice cream when I had my mother with me. We sat at a picnic bench among the crew and ate a dish of vanilla ice cream. They were very interested in hearing about our experience and observations over the past 12 hours.

We arrived at Jackie's two-bedroom apartment just shy of midnight after an 18-hour evacuation. It was a pleasure and a relief to see her. Jackie greeted us warmly. We told her that we were very happy to see her and very glad that she could host us.

My mother had remained awake the entire trip. In fact, on more than one occasion I woke to the words, "James, are you falling asleep?" (Driving at ten miles an hour for ten hours would make any driver sleepy.)

Jackie gave us her bedroom with the queen-size bed which I shared with my mother. She took the spare room. Jackie stayed with us, listening to me describe the evacuation, while I prepared my mother for bed. We all were asleep by 1 a.m.

I woke the next morning about 8 a.m. when I heard the door open and close. Jackie had departed to walk her dog. We stayed for three days as her guest while we waited to hear that power had been restored in Clear Lake, and that conditions were safe to return. Our time with Jackie was a gift for me. I so much enjoyed watching these two cousins who had known each other for more than 75 years interact: touching, hugging, chatting, smiling, laughing.

The drive back to Clear Lake was a breeze. We drove the speed limit, and arrived after just under five hours. At home, there was no noticeable damage. Our community had power and water. I cooked pasta for dinner, and we had fresh fruit for dessert. We both were tired from the trip, and went to bed early.

Two days later the NASA Johnson Space Center re-opened. The opening was delayed because many of the astronauts and NASA staff lived in neighborhoods that still did not have power, and they were unable to return. Deborah and I had an unexpected vacation from which we were happy to have returned safely and without incident.

When I reread the description of events up until now in this chapter, it seems as if much of my mother's time with me was difficult, troublesome, even life-threatening. There were five different home health-care aides who served six separate periods of duty caring for my mother; two hospitalizations during which one major operation was performed; the deaths of Sheba and Gizmo who had been our loving companions for almost eight years; two physical attacks during which my mother had been directly in harm's way; and a massive hurricane which destroyed entire neighborhoods only a few miles away from us.

Despite all that, we thrived on the many the fun events which Clear Lake and Houston offered us. Between Galveston, 18 miles south and downtown Houston, 18 miles north, we participated in all forms of entertainment, many of which were free.

At Galveston, there was no cost to walk stretches of the beach. Maneuvering the wheelchair through the soft sand sometimes was a challenge for me, but the chair glided easily over the hard sand at the water's edge. Along the beach wall, across the street from the San Luis Resort, were dozens of tourist traps and a few good restaurants which offered "fresh catch" seafood. My mother's favorite restaurant was IHOP where she always ate crepes and drank coffee.

In Clear Lake, only two miles from our home was Armand Bayou Nature Center. At 2,500 acres, it is the largest urban wilderness preserve in the United States. The Nature Center is home to more than 370 species of birds, mammals, reptiles, and amphibians. More than 220 species of birds visit using the center to rest during their migratory journeys. Armand Bayou Nature Center lies along the Central Flyway which is the largest migratory bird route in North America. Absent the mosquitoes, or when toting plenty of bug spray, it is a great place to be outdoors.

Kemah Boardwalk, in Nassau Bay, only seven miles away, hosts an amusement park, shops and several pubs and restaurants, three of which are on the water. When the weather was warm, we would take lunch outdoors at the waterside, shielding our food from marauding sea gulls always eager to dive and snatch something away from inattentive diners. Thursday evenings, beginning at 5 p.m., live bands would perform. My mother enjoyed people-watching as many of the locals and tourists danced and socialized.

Neither of us ever cared much for the music.

Nothing generated more laughs for her than watching T-ball baseball practices and games. The children, just learning the fundamentals of baseball, outperformed television's *The Little Rascals* for spontaneous comedy. Some of the boys were so small that they were shorter than the stand on which the ball rested. These squeakers had to swing at an awkward, upward angle and often missed the ball. But strikes never were called and the young athletes kept trying until they got a hit. Sometimes the batter ran to first base, sometimes he ran to third base. Often, he looked to his coach or his father to show him which way to run. A hit, not much more than a bunt, brought in the entire infield to grab the ball. Where the ball was thrown after it was snatched was anybody's guess. But certainly, it never was thrown to whatever base, position or teammate the thrower had intended as his target.

The players' uniforms were at least two sizes too big. The same was true for the baseball caps. Most of the fielders used gloves that were three times the size of their little hands. If a ball rolled in a fielder's direction, he tended to use the glove as a big scooper, trapping it with one hand and holding it in place with the other.

Less than two miles from our home is Clear Lake High School with a student population of approximately 2,500 in grades 9 through 12.

The high school boasts a full orchestra, a full marching band, a wind ensemble, a choir, and a theater department all of which have won awards for achievement throughout Texas and the United States.

Every year the theater department would host a play in which members of the senior class performed. The entrance fee was only $10, waived for my mother given her status. We attended every play, preferring the Sunday matinee at 3 p.m. for convenience. We always arrived early so that I could secure an aisle seat for my mother and a seat next to her for me.

Without exception, each of the plays was sensational. Our favorite was *Footloose.* The music was exceptional and the dancing was also. After the performance, my mother and I congratulated the cast, the male and female dancers still sweating profusely after their powerful dance routines.

We also attended the concerts by the band, orchestra and choir. On our street there were neighbors whose children performed in both groups. Ricky's daughter Jessie was a member of the band. Most of the music my mother recognized, especially song and dance tunes from the 30's, 40's and 50's, and songs from various musicals.

In the spring of each year, the school district of which we were a part, hosts an annual Senior to Senior Prom. Seniors, age 60 or older are treated to an evening of dinner and dancing by the seniors from the graduating class of the district's high schools: Clear Brook, Clear Creek, Clear Falls, Clear Horizons, Clear Lake, Clear Springs and Clear View. The seniors help decorate, serve dinner and join their special guests, folks 50 years or more senior to them, out on the dance floor. Although my mother no longer could dance, she always could eat and enjoy the music. The Senior to Senior Prom is sponsored by local businesses.

"Houston, the Eagle has landed." (From the voice of Neil Armstrong at 4:18 p.m. on July 20, 1969, when the Apollo 11 lunar lander touched down on the moon.)

"Houston, we have a problem." (A comment by astronaut Jack Swigert and echoed somewhat similarly by astronaut James A. Lovell following an explosion onboard the Apollo 13 spacecraft.)

Who, except folks from the oil industry, would know anything about Houston if not for NASA's Johnson Space Center and the astronaut community which resides there?

During my time as an employee with NASA at the Johnson Space Center, astronauts launched aboard a Space Shuttle from the Kennedy Space Center in Florida to serve on short-duration Space Shuttle missions (an average of 10 days), or longer duration missions (as long as six months) on the International Space Station (ISS). Astronauts also launched aboard a Soyuz platform from Baikonur, Russia to serve missions of varying lengths on the ISS.

At the end of these missions, the Shuttle and Station crews always returned to Ellington Field where they were met by their families, the NASA teams which supported their missions, and the public. At every return, a NASA Flight Director or Mission Manager would welcome home the crew, explain the highlights of the mission, and then each member of the crew would describe his or her experience.

My job as a NASA engineer was to identify, design, construct, test, validate and manifest science and engineering experiments, primarily from Europe, universities, and the United States military, for demonstration on the Space Shuttle and Space Station. During my 11 years with NASA in Clear Lake, I attended every return of the crew including the historic return from the final flights of Space Shuttles Discovery, Endeavour and Atlantis. My mother attended with me for the 10 years that we were together. She met and knew many of the astronauts. Eight would attend her funeral in February 2010.

The crew returns were popular events that always were crowded. But we had attended so often that the NASA support staff at Ellington Field reserved a parking place for our vehicle and an aisle position for us within the restricted area for the crew families and their guests. My mother always was attentive and joined in the frequent applause at the arrival and welcome and during the Welcome Home ceremony and mission review.

Usually within three to six weeks after

the crew return, NASA would host a second mission briefing and awards ceremony in the auditorium at Space Center Houston, a huge tourist facility located across from the Johnson Space Center. We attended those also. The parking fee was waved for me as a NASA-badged employee. NASA also provided my mother a "Support Member" badge that she wore on a lanyard around her neck at all the crew returns and awards ceremonies. It was not unusual for members of the crew to recognize us and greet her when we crossed paths at places and events within the Clear Lake community.

In addition to these many fun (and free) activities, there were numerous other annual events and festivals which, weather permitting, also were fun and entertaining.

My mother's grandmother emigrated from Ireland to the United States in the mid-1800's. It was only natural that St. Patrick's Day in March should attract us two Irish-something Catholics to the celebrations.

Dressed in green, we attended our first festival in downtown Houston hosted by one of the Catholic churches. It was a disaster. There was no parking anywhere close to the festival area. I had to push the wheelchair over cobblestone sidewalks from which there were no cutouts to the sidewalks to enable wheelchairs to cross the streets. When we arrived at the festival, all the seating in the shade was taken. There restroom facilities were all inside the church and accessible only by stairs. We left immediately and drove to a local restaurant. We ate the traditional meal of corned beef and cabbage. My mother drank ice tea and had a couple of sips from my mug of green beer.

The next year we drove in the opposite direction to Galveston where the festival was doubly as miserable as the one a year earlier in Houston. In Galveston, the festival was held on a blocked-off street. There was no parking anywhere in the area, even for someone traveling in a vehicle with a handicapped-designated license plate. Moving the wheelchair on the sidewalks and streets among folks who had far too much to drink by 11 a.m. was a threat to my mother's safety. The music was too loud and the lines for the food were too long. Again, we opted to celebrate in a restaurant. We went back to the San Luis Resort.

On our third attempt we hit a home run at a place I should have gone to the first time: The American Legion, Post 490, Ellington Field. It has the largest membership in the United States. I had been a member of the American Legion since 1979 when I joined in the Canal Zone, Panama. Tammy, my mother's hairdresser worked there as a bartender. I never thought of it. Once I started caring for my mother, I never visited the Post.

Inside there was a band playing Irish tunes. Two male Legionnaire drinking buddies offered us their table which we gladly accepted. The

$10.00 buffet offered all-you-can-eat bowls of Irish stew, plates of corned beef, cabbage and carrots, cake with green icing and mint chocolate chip ice cream. We missed not seeing Tammy. But it was a wonderful St. Patrick's Day celebration. We returned every year and sat at a table which Tammy and the management had reserved for us.

The next month, usually in early April, NASA hosted an annual Chili Cook Off competition, at a large grassy field on site at the Johnson Space Center. Beginning at 7 a.m., teams of any size would begin to set-up their cook sites and start to prepare what each team thought was the best chili in Texas, probably in the United States and possibly in the world.

Visitors could buy tickets which enabled them to judge "storefronts" and vote for the "Best Chili." During the day there were games for the children and a Space Trivia Contest for the space geeks.

At noon, teams needed enough chili available for the official judges and ticket holders to begin tasting the chili. At 2 p.m. the judges ended their testing and made their decisions which ranked the teams; at 3 p.m. the "people's choice" votes were tallied and teams ranked again. An awards ceremony was held at 4:30 p.m., and the Cook Off ended after the ceremony.

My mother and I attended every year that the

weather cooperated, usually arriving at noon and departing after about two hours. Chili never was a staple in my mother's diet for a variety of reasons. We each sampled probably no more than what would amount to a cereal-bowl size of chili. It was more fun for us to circulate among the teams, many members who we knew from my work, and the visitors, many of whom we knew from our neighborhood. They all were very kind to us, some folks bringing my mother a sample of the chili. "Here, Miss Dorothy. This may be a winner. Enjoy."

For more than 20 years an annual "Clear Lake Greek Festival," sponsored by the local St. John the Theologian Greek Orthodox Church, was held in Clear Lake Park, only one mile east of the Johnson Space Center. It almost always was held on Mothers' Day weekend in mid-May.

The church sponsors bragged that "This festival again will bring the aromas, sounds, tastes and traditions of Greece to the Clear Lake area." Certainly it did. Tickets were inexpensive. Seating was at large, shared tables. The food was served buffet style.

We would arrive shortly before noon. I always was lucky to find a corner position at a table close to the stage where my mother could enjoy a meal and watch the performers. The dancers of both sexes all were dressed in traditional Greek costumes. They performed in four groups: adults, mid-teens and 20's, grade- and middle-school-age children, and everyone all together.

Only about two miles away from the home

where my family lived on Long Island was a very popular, but small, Greek restaurant with great food at a good price. Meals were served with a complimentary glass of Greek wine. My parents visited almost weekly after they had retired and their children had moved away. I'm sure that it was there that my mother developed her taste for Greek cuisine.

Every year that we attended the festival, I always was surprised at how much food my mother could consume at one sitting, including two, sometimes three, Greek-specialty desserts, while she watched the dancers. It made me wonder if I were not feeding her enough at home. Or maybe it was the dose of "filoxenia" (Greek hospitality and spirit) which sparked her appetite.

Following the Greek Festival in the third week of May, occasionally coinciding with my mother's birthday on the 20th, is the annual, three-day Pasadena Strawberry Festival. It is a tradition going back more than 40 years.

Deborah had lived in Pasadena before she lost her home after Billy's death. She would pass by the 106-acre Pasadena Fairgrounds, at which the festival was held, on her way to and from our home. Pasadena, Texas had once been known as the "Strawberry Capital of the South," producing tons of strawberries loaded on to train cars for distribution nationally. Over time, the strawberry fields were replaced by oil fields after the petro-chemical companies discovered the area.

Weather permitting, on one of the three days, perfect if that day were her birthday, we would drive to the festival, arriving late-morning. On occasion, we were lucky to arrive in time to view the Opening Day Festival Parade.

There was much more than just strawberries to see, sample and eat. Young athletes and older pretend-athletes of both sexes competed in 16 regulation-size pits to play mud-volleyball. The pits were dug into the soil, which at one time held strawberries, and filled with three feet of water. Over the weekend, more than 100 teams competed for the first-place trophy. The festival also had a carnival, BBQ cook-off, helicopter rides, and more than 250 vendors selling food and various items which no one would need for anything, at any time or anywhere.

We enjoyed watching the strawberry-eating contests for adults and children (they were the most fun), pig races, strolling acts, magic shows and jugglers. My mother especially enjoyed watching the toddlers at the pony rides and petting zoo.

There were three stages for entertainment. Performances started at noon and ended when the festival closed for the day. My impression was that most of the bands had one or two musicians and two or three noisemakers. Except for a soloist or a band belting out some Country-Western music, the rest of what we heard was only noise. After three or four hours, we returned home having exhausted our daily capacity for fun, travel and adventure.

Without exception, the most satisfying form of entertainment for us was a performance at Jones Hall, home to the Houston Symphony Orchestra and the Society for the Performing Arts. Located in downtown Houston, Jones Hall was a 25-mile, relatively-easy drive from our home. Matinees were at 2 p.m. Evening performance were at 7:30 p.m. or 8 p.m.

We started our drive there 90 minutes ahead of the time scheduled for the performance. Arriving early, after about a 40-minute drive, ensured that I would find one of only about a dozen handicapped parking spaces located in an underground garage adjacent to an entrance into the Hall. After arrival, we would move from the vehicle to a small, park-like area between the garage and the entrance where there were two wrought iron tables, each with four chairs, and a fish pond with a splash fountain. The area was bordered by trimmed, green hedges aligned behind seasonal multi-colored plants.

At one of the tables, both of which always were unoccupied, (the few early-arrival concert-goers preferring the glamour of the interior with its first-class bar and bistro), I served our dinner. First, I seated my mother on a chair, made more comfortable by the padded cushion from her wheelchair. Then I returned to the SUV from which I retrieved a cooler. From it, I took and set on the table a linen tablecloth, two plates, silverware, water glasses, and two vases each containing small cuttings of blooming Alstroemeria. The meal was simple: brie and crackers, a few slices of roasted chicken, macaroni salad, and grapes. Ice cream always melted in the cooler so I substituted fruit yogurt for dessert. We drank iced tea, poured cold from a thermos into the water glasses. We finished in about half an hour, giving me another 30 minutes before the performance to clear the table, return the cooler, make a stop at one of the handicapped restrooms and take our seats.

Seating within the massive Jones Hall was spacious. My mother and I always sat in an extra-wide row designed specifically for handicapped persons, especially those who used wheelchairs. The row was designated "Orchestra" and was located about 20 rows away from the stage. It was so wide and easily accessible that individuals using motorized wheelchairs could drive down the aisle and parallel park into a space large enough for their wheelchairs. The seats were ordered with an open space to accommodate someone seated in a wheelchair of any type and with a standard theater-size companion seat next to it. This arrangement was then re-created in a mirror image so that it formed a pod of four spaces: two wheelchair places, one at each end, and two companion seats next to each other in the center of the pod.

I always transferred my mother from her wheelchair into the companion seat where I had added her padded cushion. It made the seat more comfortable and gave her a few more inches of elevation to view the performance somewhat better. I sat in the wheelchair.

Often, there were looks of surprise by late-comers who had not seen me transfer my mother to her seat, but did see me stand up from the wheelchair and walk, obviously not disabled, to greet someone whom we knew.

We attended 34 performances in just under 10 years. The performers never failed to dazzle us and the audience.

We were thrilled by the songs from entertainers such as Paul Anka, Burt Bacharach, Tony Bennett, Glen Campbell (Helen attended with us), The Chieftains, Marvin Hamlisch, Eileen Ivers, Anne Murray and the Preservation Hall Jazz.

Usually, the performances began with an introductory theme song which the orchestra played as the curtain slowly opened. At the end of the song, Houston Symphony Conductor Mike Krajewski would turn to face the audience, welcome everyone, thank them for their attendance and support of the Symphony, and describe the highlights for the evening's performance. Then he would turn again and the concert would begin. The entertainer would enter from one side of the stage, then move to center-stage as the audience applauded.

But the concert by Paul Anka had a very different and very surprising start. The orchestra began playing one of his more famous songs, *Diana*, behind a closed curtain. As the curtain opened, Mr. Anka entered not from one side of the stage but from the door to our right. He began singing as he started walking the length of the extra-wide handicapped aisle. He would sing part of a verse,

I'm so young and you're so old

This, my darling, I've been told

I don't care just what they say

Cause forever I will pray

while stopping in front of the first pod and shaking hands with the four persons seated there.

Moving down the aisle,

You and I will be as free

As the birds up in the trees

Oh, please stay by me, Diana

another pause, and another four persons awe-struck as Paul Anka shook their hands.

Continuing to move and sing now the second verse,

Thrills I get when you hold me close

Oh, my darling, you're the most

I love you but do you love me

Oh, Diana, can't you see

he stopped directly in front of us.

I love you with all my heart

And I hope we will never part

Oh, please stay with me, Diana

He shook hands with the couple to our right and then reached for my mother's hand as she offered it. But each was unable to break the vise-clamp grip which my mother had on Paul Anka's hand. He continued singing as he looked quickly at me and I said, "Mr. Anka, she has Parkinson's disease. I have to open her hand."

He gave me a quick nod and stood locked hand in hand with my mother while he finished the first part of the third verse:

Oh, my darlin', oh, my lover

` Tell me that there is no other

I love you with all my heart

Oh-oh, oh-oh, oh-oh

It was during the "Oh-oh, oh-oh, oh-oh," that I leaned forward, gestured as if I now were adding my hand to theirs, and broke the grip.

He finished the rest of the third verse moving to the end of the aisle, and the final part on the stage. At the intermission, people came to us asking, "How do you know Paul Anka? Are you all family? Is it possible you could get his autograph for us?" I can't remember what I said to all of these people. My mother

302

took it all in stride, sitting in her chair and smiling at everyone. I let some folks pet her shoulders and arms. I remained standing and holding her right hand to keep the secret of our relationship with Paul Anka between my mother and me.

The Symphony performed several specialized concerts such as Modern Broadway, Club Swing, Gershwin: An American Original, Irish Pops, and Pops Knockouts. Following the re-entry disintegration of Space Shuttle Columbia on February 1, 2003, the Symphony recognized the seven-member crew, their families and the Houston community with a free performance four days later on February 5th, entitled "The Columbia Memorial Concert." Willie McCool, pilot for the Columbia, was one of the astronauts who played poker at my home with the NASA engineers who supported his training and this mission. He told us that, beyond being an astronaut, his true claim to fame was defeating President George W. Bush in a race at a school track meet in Texas.

Each year at Jones Hall ended for us with two concerts in December to celebrate Christmas. The first, in mid-December was "A Very Merry Pops," at the end of which the audience sang songs of the season along with Mike Krajewski and the members of the orchestra. The second, within a week of Christmas Day, was the powerful "Handel's Messiah," reverent, spiritual and inspirational.

At the end of the evening performances, around 10 p.m., we would wait until most of the audience had departed before we exited. Then we would move to one of the handicapped restrooms for the last time of the evening to tend to my mother's hygiene. On the drive home, still very much wide awake, I would watch her look past me at the Golden Arches as we approached the local McDonald's only a half mile from home. It never was too late to drive through, order and enjoy a dish of plain vanilla ice cream which we ate while parked across the street on the campus of the University of Houston, Clear Lake.

These concerts served as revivals for my mother's spirit. They brought out the life that was still within her but was masked by the effects of her Parkinson's disease.

The year 2009 was our final year as concert-goers to Jones Hall. In December, the Creator gave my mother her two favorite Christmas concerts there and a very Merry Christmas at our home with her family and friends.

Not too long after the start of the new year, my mother began a slow, but noticeable, decline. She slept longer through the night and napped more frequently during the day. Her appetite declined considerably. The volume of pureed foods which she was able to consume started to decrease slowly. Her eyes closed often when we would feed and bathe her, unless we tried to start and maintain a simple conversation. Even then it was hard for her to remain attentive. It also was difficult for Deborah and me to keep her engaged in any activity. We decided that it would be more peaceful for her if we stayed close so that she could sense our presence, but did not try to coerce her to do anything other than eat.

Toward the end of January, the 27th being the 14th anniversary of the death of her husband and the 29th being their 60th wedding anniversary, I called Carmel and asked for her help. She came immediately to our home, spoke with Deborah and me, then sat alone and spoke with my mother. Carmel told me, "Jim, I'm sure you sense that the end is near. You may have only a few more weeks with your mother. I think that you should call your sisters. And for now, you and Deborah should just do the simple things that will keep your mother comfortable."

I had been planning to do that. Carmel gave me the encouragement. I spoke first with Janet, and later with Kathy. I suggested that we speak daily in the evenings when I could update them on our mother's status.

During the first week of February, my mother decreased the volume of food she consumed by half. During the second week, she stopped eating completely. Deborah and I were able to get her only to swallow some chilled applesauce and drink some iced tea or water. Toward the end of the second week in February, it was difficult for her to accept a straw and to swallow any fluids.

Kathy and Janet arrived just before the start of the three-day President's Day weekend. I had a very difficult time watching my sisters try to interact with our mother, knowing that these last days with her were at least as difficult for them as they were for me. Perhaps it was a time of peace for them. But in no way was it a pleasant experience.

One of my sisters suggested that I call our parish priest, which I did. Father Bob arrived at our home on Monday, February 15th, the Presidents' Day holiday, to administer the last rites, now referred to as the Sacrament of Healing or the Anointing of the Sick.

Father Bob stood in front of our mother who was reclining on the sofa. My sisters and I stood behind or to the side of the sofa facing him. We recited the prayers which he led.

For the last five years of her life, the muscle rigidity caused by the Parkinson's had the effect of locking her elbows against her sides, forcing her forearms and hands to be crossed stiffly against her chest, and locking her fingers into tight fists. When I would bathe her, I would have to peel back each arm to it and one side of her body. I also would have to pry open her fingers and quickly place a washcloth or small bar of soap onto the palm of her hand to wash her hand and fingers. As soon as I stopped, her hand would snap shut.

While Father Bob recited his prayers, there was no indication that our mother had any awareness of the event. But as Father Bob anointed her forehead, drawing with his thumb the sign of the cross and saying the words, "I absolve you in the name of the Father, Son, . . ." my mother turned her head toward him, opened her eyes and hands, then raised her outstretched arms and hands as if to embrace him. After Father Bob concluded the Anointing, my mother closed her eyes and lowered her arms back to her sides.

Slowly her body relaxed. All the rigidity from the Parkinson's receded like a wave from the shore. The pale, clammy appearance of her face was transformed to a soft rosy blush. The specs of calcium deposits which sprinkled isolated parts of her body evaporated. My two sisters and I were amazed. What had we four just witnessed?

The rigidity never returned. Mother's arms, hands and fingers remained as flexible as if she never had been affected by Parkinson's disease. When Deborah came to visit, she was as surprised by the transformation as we were.

The next day, Tuesday, February 16th, Carmel visited again. One of my sister's sat on the sofa with our mother holding and massaging her legs on her lap. Carmel sat on a chair close to my mother's upper body and kept her thumb on her pulse. My other sister and I stood close by. No one did much talking. The silence was interrupted only when Carmel looked at me and said calmly, "Jim, she's gone." We all were overwhelmed with emotion.

Dorothy Muriel Hyacinth Rinderknecht Pelosi died at 5:10 p.m., Tuesday, February 16, 2010. She was three months shy of her 86th birthday.

Carmel continued to offer her support as she took her leave from the family. I recovered well enough to call the family doctor and inform him. His staff contacted the funeral parlor.

My sense of loss was intensified when I watched the funeral parlor staff remove my mother from the sofa, place her on a gurney, wheel her out the front door, and lift her into the hearse. The vehicle drove to the end of the cul-de-sac, turned around and drove past the house. I waved "Goodbye." I could not come to grips with the events of this final departure.

I was very surprised when I read the "Cause of Death" at the Death Certificate. It read: "malnutrition, dehydration." It made me feel as if I had killed my mother. But then I remembered what I wrote earlier in this narrative at Chapter 2, *"What is this Disease,"* that a person does not die from Parkinson's disease but with Parkinson's disease. Still, it did not make me feel any better.

Four days later, a funeral Mass was held at our parish church. Father Dominic and Father Bob co-celebrated the Mass. Mrs. Carmel Garan and Mrs. Arlene Cooley, a very good friend and coworker at NASA, recited the readings. Following the gospel, I spoke the eulogy.

That day, I was so very proud of my mother and my sisters knowing how much we had accomplished as a family. I was also very proud and thankful for the support my family received from our friends, neighbors and the professionals who helped care for her and who attended her funeral. I remain especially grateful to my NASA coworkers and the eight astronauts who, given their demanding pre-flight training schedules, also attended the funeral with their families.

My mother is interred together with my father at the South Florida Veterans Cemetery in Lake Worth, Florida.

The inscription on her side of the tombstone reads:

P E L O S I

D O R O T H Y   R

MAY 20, 1924 – FEBRUARY 16, 2010

NO GREATER LOVE

DEVOTED WIFE

BELOVED MOTHER

Upon reflection, almost nine years after my mother's death, I do not know how I managed for 10 years to maintain the routine, where I got the energy to do all the work, and why I almost never felt tired. I know I never was sick. I suffered only a detached retina as a result of an airborne collision while playing basketball, but that changed nothing. I had a similar level of activity and energy for 30 years while I was in the Army and serving with all branches of the military. My sentiment is that anyone with a sense of dedication and passion about anything, especially something that involves other people, derives the energy naturally. Certainly, that was true for me with my soldiers when I served with them in the Army and with my mother when I cared for her at our home.

"Blessed are they who hunger and thirst for righteousness, for they will be satisfied."

A Beatitude, adapted from Matthew's description of the Sermon on the Mount.

15. RISE UP!

Our Senior Citizens.

The word, "righteousness" has several inherent characteristics which help to understand fully its meaning. They are decency, honesty, justice, morality, and virtue. In this chapter I try to describe the extent of my outrage at the current healthcare system in the United States and my righteous goal for the reform of Medicare to fund the essential care which all senior citizens require as they age. The reform I seek and will work for would provide sustaining quality-of-life care for our senior citizens which presently is not funded by Medicare.

I believe my sources information to be true and my comments follow from that belief. This chapter is intended to help lessen one of the greatest evils facing senior citizens in the United States today, that of the lack of taxpayer-funded care to provide for necessities directly associated with aging: dental exams and care; eye exams, care and supplies; and hearing exams, care and supplies.

I am reminded much too often of my parents and their two siblings. The bread winners worked at their jobs until retirement. While they worked, they and their spouses raised seven children; sent those children to public or parochial schools through the 12th grade, and then to colleges or universities where they earned their degrees. These seniors owned their own homes. They owned their own automobiles. They paid their taxes without delinquency. They bought much with cash and little with credit. They respected the law. My parents never had as much as a traffic ticket. I assume that the same would be true for my two uncles and two aunts.

When they all reached age 65, they became eligible for Medicare.

Medicare did not cover their vision care services such as routine eye exams for eyeglasses or contact lenses or absorb the cost of eyeglasses or contact lenses which they may have needed. In the absence of any insurance for which they may have paid a premium, they paid for this from their own funds.

Medicare did not cover routine hearing exams or fittings for hearing aids or absorb the cost of hearing aids which they may have needed. In the absence of any insurance for which they may have paid a premium, they paid for this from their own funds.

Medicare did not cover routine dental exams or dental care and procedures such as cleanings, fillings, tooth extractions, dentures, dental plates, or other dental devices. In the absence of any insurance for which they may have paid a premium, they paid for this from their own funds.

I think that there is not a single American citizen over the age of 18 who does not have the awareness that all persons require dental exams and dental care to maintain their health throughout their lives; that most senior citizens wear eyeglasses; and, that many senior citizens use hearing aids.

The United States is the richest, most productive and most technologically advanced and energetic country in the world, and has been. In the 1920's the United States was supplying beer to Germany, pottery to Bohemia and oranges to Valencia.

Today, in 2019, global Gross Domestic Product (GDP) is approximately 75 trillion U.S. dollars. The United States alone contributes approximately 13.5 trillion dollars, about 18 percent. In Fiscal Year 2018, the United States government collected approximately 1.7 trillion dollars in taxes.

Exams, eyeglasses, hearing aids and dental care are not a personal issue for members of the U.S. Congress, for the wealthy, for many persons who are imprisoned, or for most of the illegals living in this country whose care is funded by Medicaid. Grandma and Grandpa go without subsidized care so that Congress and the criminals (is there a difference?) can have it.

What do the numbers say?

"FAIR" (The Federation for American Immigration Reform) contends that between $11 billion to $22 billion is spent on welfare to illegal immigrants annually by state governments. A national media source states that the American taxpayer funds $90 billion annually for welfare and social services to illegal immigrants.

"CIS" (The Center for Immigration Studies) states that $22 billion a year is spent on Food Assistance programs such as food stamps, "WIC" (Special Supplemental Nutrition Program for Women, Infants, and Children which provides healthcare and nutrition for low-income pregnant women, breastfeeding women, and children under the age of five), and free lunches at schools for illegal immigrants. Additional information from CIS asserts that $2.5 billion a year is spent on Medicaid for illegal immigrants.

Information from "transcripts.cnn.com" reports that $17 billion a year is spent for the education of children born in the United States to illegal immigrant parents. These children are referred to by the media and others as "anchor babies."

The cost to incarcerate illegal immigrants, who make up approximately 30 percent of the USA Federal prison population, is estimated by the government at about $3 million a day.

These costs alone amount to $155 billion which represents taxpayer dollars not spent on those senior citizens for the essentials they need as they continue to age. Presently, the "Baby Boomer" generation, of which I am a member, is the fastest growing age group in the United States. As of 2018, 14.5 percent of the nation's population was age 65 or older. In 10 years, in 2029, the national population of those age 65 or older will increase to 20 percent.

Why am I not surprised?

The following represents the annual revenue in 2017 for the 10 largest Health Care providers in the United States:

1. McKessan Corporation*, San Francisco, California: $208.3 billion.
   * McKesson is the oldest and largest healthcare company in the nation.

2. United Health Group*, Minnetonka, Minnesota: $201.0 billion.
   *Also a Health Insurance Plan (HIP) provider.

3. CVS Health, Woonsocket, Rhode Island: $184.7 billion.

4. AmerisourceBergen Corporation*, Chesterbrook, Pennsylvania: $153.1 billion.
*Parent Company for Walgreens and Express Scripts which accounted for 45 percent of its 2017 annual revenue.

5. Cardinal Health, Dublin, Ohio: $129.9 billion.

6. Express Scripts Holding, St. Louis, Missouri* #: $100.6 billion
*As of 2018, the company is the 25th-largest in the United States by total revenue. It is the largest pharmacy benefit management organization in the United States.
#Prescription drug delivery accounted for 98 percent of its 2017 annual revenue.

7. Anthem, Inc.*, Indianapolis, Indiana: $89.1 billion.
*Also a Health Insurance Plan (HIP) provider.

8. Kaiser Permanente, Oakland, California: $72.7 billion.

9. Aetna*, Hartford, Connecticut: $63 billion.
*A Health Insurance Plan (HIP) provider.

10. Humana*, Louisville, Kentucky: $54.3 billion.
*Also a Health Insurance Plan (HIP) provider.

The following represents the annual revenue in 2017 for the seven largest Pharmaceutical Companies in the United States:

1. Pfizer, New York City, New York: $52.5 billion.

2. Johnson and Johnson, New Brunswick, New Jersey: $36.3 billion.

3. Merck & Company, Kenilworth, New Jersey: $35.4 billion.

4. AbbVie, North Chicago, Illinois: $28.2 billion.

5. Gilead, Foster City, California: $25.6 billion.

6. Amgen, Inc, Thousand Oaks, California: $22.8 billion.

Among the highest paid Chief Executive Officers (CEO's) in the United States are:

- Johnson and Johnson's Alex Gorsky at $22.995,564.

- Aetna's Mark Bertolini at $18, 702,992. (Aetna, above, #9 at "largest Health Care providers in the United States.)

Television Commercials.

I have a very strong bias against television which my parents referred to as "the idiot box." I owned a television when I lived in the United States to support the occasional visits by my family and friends. But I never watched television alone. I never owned a television for the 18 years that I served overseas with the military and various agencies of the United States government.

Before my mother came to live with me in Houston, my NASA coworkers, who visited to play poker, bought me a wide-screen television. I had scheduled a poker game on the same night as of one of the championship basketball games, and they wanted to watch or listen to it while they were taking my money. I gave away the television after my mother died.

I don't watch sports; I play them. I don't watch history programs; I read. I don't watch travel or nature shows; I take trips and explore. Television news is abhorrent. In the United States, but not in Europe, in hotel breakfast rooms I'm subjected to noise about murders, rapes, molestations, politics, traffic wrecks and weather 1,000 miles from where I'm staying before I've had my first cup of coffee. Televisions are everywhere: airports, bars, hospitals, medical offices, nursing homes, and restaurants. There even is an idiot box at gasoline pumps.

When I volunteer to work at a hospital, Veterans Affairs (VA) clinic or care facility, I'm forced to listen to the television while I'm supporting a patient. Commercials dominate the broadcasts. Most of them, start with the words, "Do you have Medicare?" They urge viewers to "ask your doctor about (Insert the name of some unpronounceable medication), or some form of equipment: back support, knee pads, neck brace, chair lift, easy-access bathtub. "Medicare pays. You pay nothing." Really? Who pays Medicare? There is a premium for Medicare deducted monthly from my Social Security check.

The most annoying part of these broadcasts are the disclaimers at the end of the commercials for medication. "Do not take 'Poppypilluppychuck' if you are a patient in an Intensive Care Unit; if you are scheduled for brain surgery; if you've had recent multiple amputations; if you've had thoughts of killing yourself, your spouse, your children, your employer, your coworkers, Santa Claus, or others; if you hear voices; have problems urinating; are constipated, have stomach pains, nausea, diarrhea; are pregnant, depressed, underweight, overweight, obese, tired, hungry, confused, easily distracted, insecure, psychotic, in debt, cannot parallel park; have had a history of alcohol or drug abuse; or enjoy attending free-lunch seminars sponsored by insurance agents or wealth management advisors."

Television viewers suffer through two minutes of "Stop what you're doing, and call your doctor or the number at the bottom of your screen now," followed by three minutes of noise which is at least equally as offensive.

Who is responsible for these "get help quick" ads? The answer is simple: all those healthcare, health insurance, and pharmaceutical companies listed above at "*why am I not surprised*?" and at least as many other health-care-related companies. They constantly prey on people, mostly seniors, who truly are sick or disabled or who fear becoming so. The sentiment is much akin to huge roadside billboards which read, "Jesus Saves." On television, it's "Medication Saves." How else can anyone explain the incredible wealth of all those companies?

In exceptional cases, medication should be the remedy of last resort.

Aging and Needing Assistance.

Until they died, my great-grandparents were cared for in the larger of their two daughters two homes. Both women shared the work and the expenses.

Three of my four grandparents died before they needed care; my grandmother lived a very healthy life to age 89. She died shortly after my father took her car away from her in response to her neighbor's complaints that she was driving too fast, not making complete stops, going out by herself to dinner and driving back home at night. Most of her life, she bought a new car every two or three years; never had an accident; never had a traffic ticket. Her death certificate reads, "Cause of death. Natural causes." I wonder what really killed her.

Earlier I wrote that I am a member of the Baby Boomer generation, those persons born between 1946 and 1965. Now, in 2019, we range in age between 54 and 73 years old.

We are followed by Generation X, those persons born between 1966 and 1980. Now, in 2019, they range in age between 39 and 53 years old.

They are followed by the Millennials, those persons born between 1981 and 1966. Now, in 2019, they range in age between 23 and 38 years old.

I retired in 2012 after working for 42 years. Members of Generation X, who had earned a four-year degree, came into the workforce around 1987. For almost 25 years I watched more and more women join that workforce. I also saw hundreds of new mothers place their infants and toddlers into day care so that they could continue working. Some of those infants were enrolled as early as eight weeks after their birth; most were enrolled between the ages of six and eight months; some working mothers waited until the child was a year old, rarely until the child was two.

One of my new-mother coworker engineers at NASA enrolled her infant boy in day care eight weeks after his birth. I asked her what she thought about the possibility of missing his first steps and his first words. Without hesitation she told me, "When I come home and see his first steps and later hear his first words, it will be a 'First' for me. So, what's the difference?" I've always wondered if any day care workers ever have been called, "Mommy," and any working mothers ever been called, "Miss Jenny"?

The average American child catches six colds a year. The average American child in day care catches 10.

I've told my closest family members and friends that if I had Bill Gates' money, I would be buying up land in and around those businesses with the largest number of employees in this country, and be building assisted living centers, memory care centers, nursing homes, and specialized care facilities. It seems reasonable to me that any child thrown into day care at an early age and kept there and elsewhere while his parents both worked would not be too eager to care for those parents once they came in need of care. Those parents would be whisked away to a facility as fast as their kids were whisked away to day care.

On a flight between Orlando and Los Angeles I sat in an aisle seat, starboard side, one row behind the second Emergency Exit row. Seated one row in front of the first Emergency Exit row, on the port side, was a woman in her late 20's or early 30's with two children about ages 4 and 6. The children were beyond control: fighting, yelling, running into the aisle, bouncing on their seats, everything a significant distraction for anyone within hearing range. The mother traded places with her two children at least four times during the flight.

After landing, a man who had been seated in the row opposite this family walked back near me to retrieve his carry-on bag. I said to him, "I assume you're not the father of those children who were seated opposite you."

He answered, "Those brats would not last two hours in my home. And if their mother objected, she'd be gone too. I'm surprised I didn't hear them yell back at her, 'who are you to tell us what to do? We don't know you.' Do you think that those kids, raised in day care since before they could walk and talk, have any respect for that woman? This is a perfect example of bad parenting."

I said, "Let's go into business together. We'll buy the land and build the facilities into which those kids will dump their parents the minute they need someone to care for them in their old age."

He answered as we exited the aircraft, "Great idea. If you have time, let's have a drink. I'm curious."

If the reader is a senior citizen or shortly approaching that status, I strongly suggest visiting a nursing home or assisted care living facility if you have not already done so. Look closely at everything. Inspect and smell all the rooms. Look at how the residents are dressed and what they are doing. Watch the events in the dining room before, during and after a meal is served. Watch how the residents interact during meals. Read the activities board. Watch the events and see how many residents participate. See who visits. Keep going back: in the morning, in the afternoon, at night, on weekends and on holidays. Decide quickly if such a facility is where you would want to spend the final years of your life. If so, will you be able to afford the care? If not, who will pay for it?

No one is too young to plan for the future. Sadly, the news about this is not at all encouraging. More than half of Americans do not have any retirement savings. The median American household has only $11,700 in savings, in checking accounts and money market funds. Baby Boomers have slightly more saved for retirement, with a median savings of $103,000. The average Millennial has just $1,000 saved for retirement.

I wrote earlier in Chapters 9 and 10, that "you win wars by planning to lose them." If you plan that someday you may lose your ability to care for yourself, or to obtain the care that you may need as you age so that you may live a comfortable and happy life in your retirement years, then you must act. Involve your family and your friends. Seek counseling from the many professionals and numerous local senior-support organizations which provide counseling for free.

Do not fail to act and condemn yourself to an existence that you may live to regret.

Invest in Illegals. Forget our Families.

what is this nonsense about providing refuge and sanctuary to persons who enter the United States illegally? How did the term "sanctuary city" evolve? Do American citizens and foreign non-citizens have a right to pick and choose which laws in the United States they want to obey? Is any of this supported by the Constitution of the United States? I, and a good number of the American electorate, especially, I assume, those citizens who elected Donald Trump as President of the United States, oppose all forms of illegal immigration. "Illegal" is the relevant issue in the immigration debate.

During the 2016 Presidential election campaign, people supporting illegal immigration argued that a wall would not work.

The United States is four time zones wide with very porous borders. The former Soviet Union was 11 times zones wide. Very few Soviets got out and very few others got in. Of course, no one wanted to get into the Soviet Union. But almost everyone, other than loyal Communist Party members, wanted to get out. There was a system in place, albeit not too friendly, which provided for very strict border control. It was possible for the former Soviet Union to protect its borders and its national security.

The Berlin Wall existed between August 1961 and November 1989 when the Wall fell. I lived within that walled city between 1973 and 1976 when I served with the Army's Berlin Brigade. The wall prevented East Berliners living under a communist regime from emigrating to free West Berlin. Between 1961 and 1989, more than 100,000 people attempted to escape. More than 5,000 people succeeded. Between 130 and 200 people died trying.

Twenty years after the fall of the Wall, there are people in the United States, the most technologically advanced country in the world, who argue that it is not possible to build an effective barrier on this country's southern border. But 60 years earlier, communist East Berlin, supported by East Germany and the former Soviet Union, was able to do so. The two situations are neither identical nor are they very similar, especially with respect to the size and the geography of the borders. But the issue of border security, as an element of national security, is identical.

Within the United States Congress, members who oppose the wall try to obtain influence and support by making noise not sense and by ignorance not knowledge. They distort the truth with a skill that could bend iron. The opposition seems to forget the maxim that "an elected official's first duty is to place his honor out of reach of all men." There is no honor associated with supporting illegal immigration. There is no honor associated with making noise, not sense, to buy or secure the votes of anyone or any group. Regarding the bias by the media, it seems as if the truth is whatever they can make others believe.

I speak Spanish. I started learning the language while I was a Cadet at West Point. When the Army assigned me to Panama between July 1977 and December 1979, I was able to put into practice what I had learned at the Academy. There was heightened tension in Panama in the late 1970's during the Congressional debate to ratify the Carter-Torrijos Treaty which would return the Canal Zone to Panama. I chose to live off base in a home in the town of Vera Cruz close to Howard Air Force Base to show the flag and to help reduce the tension between the locals and my unit of more than 180 soldiers. Speaking Spanish with my neighbors and in the small town helped me to do that.

I returned to Latin America and served with the Army in Honduras between 1986 and 1987 at Palmerola Air Force Base. I traveled twice monthly to brief the State Department and other United States agencies on the status of what was called, "The United States Continuing Presence in Latin America," which described security operations being conducted from Palmerola Air Force Base.

I served a third tour of duty in Latin America between 1989 and 1990 in support of Operation Just Cause which, beginning on 20

December 1989, was the action by the United States military to depose drug czar and President Manuel Noriega in Panama.

During seven years in Latin America, I visited 14 of the 20 countries to which the United States provides or provided some form of aid. To date, I have lived in seven countries for work and have visited 21 countries as a tourist. The only places where I have been food poisoned, not once but five times, (two times so severely that I required hospitalization), was during my tours of duty in Latin America. Those experiences alone, would have been motivation for me to join a caravan and sneak into the United States.

The Caravans: what's Real? What's True?

What are the reasons that so many people are fleeing their home countries, not for one of the other 19 countries within Latin America, but for Los Estados Unidos?

The migrants, their supporters, and much of the media contend that the people fleeing north are oppressed and that their countries are ravaged by violence. The media reports that El Salvador, Guatemala and Honduras are among the most violent countries in the world, plagued by dangerous gangs of drug-traffickers and other types of criminals, corrupt police and politicians on the take.

So what else is new in Latin America? How many movies has Hollywood made in the last 50 years about violence and corruption in Latin

America? How many Americans have been imprisoned there because they traveled to Latin America to find drugs?

Does anyone really know the miserable histories of most of the countries in Latin America, or do people rely on the noise by the media and the vote-hungry politicians for their information?

Remember the Hutus and Tutsis? All the violence, corruption and misery in the caravan-people countries pale in relation to the violence between these two African tribes. In 1972, in Burundi, between 80,000 and 200,000 Hutus were slaughtered by the Tutsi army. Later, in 1994, the Hutus sought revenge in Rwanda. Between 800,000 and 1 million people were killed in three months. Does anyone, especially anyone in the southern border states which are overrun by illegal immigrants, have a Hutu or Tutsi as a neighbor, someone who was granted asylum and immigration into the United States because of that extreme level of violence? I think not.

In Latin America, the oppressed in the countryside flee to the cities; those in the cities flee to the countryside. When those relocations are equally as miserable, they flee their native countries and head north.

Do the drug dealers, thieves, rapists, murderers, corrupt police and politicians, extortionists and all the other bad guys who prey on their countrymen and others all stay in their countries, content to live off their criminal behavior? I think not. Are only the kind, considerate, gentle, loving, law abiding, oppressed people longing to be free those persons who flee north? Again, I think not. Statistics which describe the prison population in the United States certainly indicate otherwise.

What about the children? It seems as if more people in more places than Vietnam took note of the impact made by photos which showed dead, maimed and orphaned children as a result of collateral damage from bombings by the United States Air Force during the Vietnam War. Those photos, and highly visible on-site protests by persons such as Hanoi Jane Fonda, were intended to sway public opinion in the United States against the war in Vietnam. Similarly, every news broadcast and every print media source do the same thing with photos of children at the border. But no mention ever is made that the sick and dying children, (two of whom have died as this is being written), never were vaccinated against illness and disease and, like their parents, or those people pretending to be their parents, are hosts for all sorts of bag bugs that make people sick.

I have written this section of the narrative, contrary to the Judeo-Christian sentiment of "Love thy Neighbor." That is not typical of my attitude and actions. Resources everywhere are limited and people everywhere must make hard choices. I choose to urge the government to reform Medicare, and to spend my tax dollars on that reform so that Medicare will pay for the costs for the dental, eye, and hearing exams, care and supplies that senior citizens will need as they age. The two relevant words in the previous sentence are "Medicare" and "citizens." I do not endorse one taxpayer dollar ever to be spent to support illegal immigration. I do support taxpayer dollars being spent to prevent illegal immigration.

Why am I so concerned about Medicare reform and the costs of illegal immigration in a narrative about Parkinson's disease? Because I believe that every senior citizen, especially those living with Parkinson's disease or other debilitating handicaps, should have the same fully-funded health care that our elected representatives have. But, because of choices made by those elected representatives about how to spend taxpayer dollars, many of the costs for senior citizen care are not fully funded by Medicare.

With respect to dental exams and dental care, Parkinson's disease can affect the mouth, teeth and jaw. The symptoms of rigidity, tremor and dyskinesia may make it difficult for a person to brush his teeth. Dry mouth is a common symptom of Parkinson's disease. It causes decreased saliva production. Saliva keeps a person's mouth wet and helps to clean the mouth by swallowing. It also contains enzymes that aid in digestion. People may experience varying degrees of dry mouth, which can impact swallowing and contribute to tooth decay and mouth infections. The reverse, the build-up of saliva, may lead to a fungal infection at the corners of the mouth. I believe that senior citizens eligible for Medicare and living with Parkinson's disease deserve Medicare-funded dental exams and dental care.

With respect to eye exams and eye care, Parkinson's disease may cause such problems as dry eyes, double vision, difficulty controlling eye movements, or other problems with the eyes and eyelids. Vision problems may affect walking and balance and result in an injury. Again, it is my opinion that senior citizens eligible for Medicare and living with Parkinson's disease deserve Medicare-funded eye exams and eye care.

Studies have confirmed a positive correlation between Parkinson's disease and hearing loss in the elderly. Those studies have shown that the decrease in dopamine in the brain has a direct correlation between hearing loss and Parkinson's disease. The research suggests that inadequate levels of dopamine, combined with age, could damage the cochlea resulting in hearing loss. Certainly, senior citizens eligible for Medicare and living with Parkinson's disease deserve Medicare-funded hearing exams, care and hearing aids if suitable.

Medicare reform first, focusing on Medicare-funded health care for all senior citizens. Medicare reform trumps (no pun intended) immigration reform. Illegal immigration never.

The Great Historical Perspectives.

I always enjoy hearing from grandparents and parents about how little history their grandchildren and children are being taught, and, even worse, learning, about American and world history, and how confused they are about what they think they know. It makes me grateful for the solid parochial- and public-school education which I received, although, after 42 years of work, I never once had to calculate the area of an isosceles triangle or quote from Caesar's *De bello Gallico.*

There is no sympathy from me for the plight of the persons in the caravans, especially the men, when the issues which they justify for fleeing their homelands are compared to the actions taken by the American colonists against the British, the Russian peasants against the Tsars, and the German officers against Hitler, all of whom faced the same or similar issues related to oppression.

The Birth of the United States of America.

America first became a British colony in 1607 when settlers arrived at Jamestown, Virginia. Many of the new colonists came to escape religious persecution, the misery of tenant farmer status, the lack of work for which they could earn and keep the wages for their labor, oppressive government controls, and other hardships which the new settlers had found intolerable.

Within the colonies, the misery of life under British control continued until it no longer could be endured. In 1765, the British passed "The Stamp Act," which was the first attempt to tax the colonists directly. Everything written or printed on paper, with the exception of private correspondence and books, would be taxed. In response, the colonists rose up and protested "no taxation without representation." Three years later, the British again inflamed the sentiments of the colonists by imposing another tax, this time on paper, tea, paint and glass.

In 1775, the members of the Continental Congress realized that reconciliation with Great Britain was unlikely. By 1776, they and the other colonists had endured enough abuse from the British. Repeated protests failed to influence or change British policies. In January 1776, the pamphlet *Common Sense*, authored by Thomas Paine, advocated independence. It was well-received and circulated widely within the colonies. Later, in the summer of 1776, the members of the Continental Congress met in Philadelphia. There, they discussed the merits of declaring independence from Great Britain. Debate began on Monday, July 1, 1776.

On Thursday, July 4, 1776, the debate ended, and the representatives of the 13 colonies voted. Twelve colonies voted for independence. New York abstained. Having renounced allegiance to King George III and Great Britain, the members of the Continental Congress formed a new nation, The United States of America.

The Declaration of Independence was read to crowds throughout Philadelphia on Monday, July 8, 1776. Because the Declaration of Independence had to be authenticated and printed, it was not signed until Friday, August 2, 1776.

King George III was not happy. He sent thousands of his trained and well-armed soldiers and sailors in hundreds of ships to suppress the colonists and defeat the revolution. Armed with only the muskets and rifles which they used to shoot squirrels for lunch and deer for supper, plus a few cannons stolen by the colonists during and after the French and Indian wars, the colonists fought back. They were aided by the French. In almost every battle, the rag-tag army of General Washington, was outnumbered, outgunned and under-supplied, yet still they fought, and fought, and fought. And they prevailed.

Six years later, under the terms of the 1783 Treaty of Paris, the "War of the American Revolution" ended. Great Britain officially acknowledged the United States as a sovereign and independent nation. The greatest military power on earth at that time had been defeated by an army of amateurs. The colonists had endured their misery from 1607 until they declared independence in 1776. The Revolutionary War ended officially in 1783.

Certainly, this victory by the persons in 13 colonies, who were motivated and allied to overcome oppression, is something that every young, able-bodied man in the caravans should recognize and understand. Turn around, go home, get organized, demonstrate and demand reform. If all that fails, revolt and fight!

The Birth of the Union of Soviet Socialist Republics.

In 1721, Peter the Great became the first emperor to rule Russia. Eight other emperors and four empresses followed him. They ruled Russia until 1917 when Vladimir Ilyich Lenin, leader of the Bolshevik Party and the October Revolution, forced Tsar Nicolas II to abdicate, seized power, and established the Soviet Union as the world's first communist state. The Bolsheviks chose comrade Lenin as their leader. Less than one year after the revolution, on July 17, 1918, Nicholas, his wife, and their five children were executed together by a firing squad.

One of the reforms promoted by the Bolsheviks was that orphans, the elderly and the disabled were to be cared for within Russian districts in specialized institutions or through subsidies.

Russia is huge, 11 time zones wide. It also is tremendously diverse. Although Russian is the only official language, there are 35 different languages which are accepted as official in the various regions. More than 100 minority languages are spoken throughout Russia. How could such a country ever be governed? How could the vast diversity of people within such a huge country fight and win World War II?

Life in Russia always was hard. A nation of peasants who lived in a servile society, its people traditionally had three major concerns: bread, land, and family. After the Tsars consolidated their empire, the peasants had two more concerns: paying taxes, and a 25-year military service obligation for males.

The discipline in the Tsars' military was draconic. The slightest infraction would be punished by flogging. After one uprising by soldiers against their commanding officer, the punishment resulted in a sentence of 6,000 lashes shared among the nine leaders (all of whom died), and the banishment to Siberia and a sentence of life at hard labor for the remaining soldiers.

Even with the majority of the peasants harboring an apolitical mentality, it did not mean that they were passive while living under a system that was based upon economic, political and social exploitation. Armed with only scythes, short-handled sickles, knives, shears, clubs, other farm tools that could be used as weapons, and occasionally firearms or explosives, the Russian peasants revolted against the Tsars 187 times before the Bolsheviks and Lenin were successful. That statement deserves repeating: the Russian peasants revolted against the Tsars 187 times before the Bolsheviks and Lenin were successful.

They stormed the Peter-Paul Fortress, used as a military base, prison and execution ground, in St. Petersburg where protesters were slaughtered by the hundreds by the Tsars' military employing light artillery, cannons, rifles with fixed bayonets and cavalry. Using the same ineffective weapons, the peasants also stormed the Tsars' palaces and government installations in Moscow where, every time, hundreds more were slaughtered by the Tsars' army and palace guards. For as long as the peasants remained subordinate to Tsarist rule, the primary reason for their oppression, backwardness and poverty, they revolted.

With this brief historical account as a second example, I again denounce the caravan trekkers, first for the cowardice of everyone capable of demanding reform and those men capable of fighting for it, and next, for their arrogance, contempt and disrespect for the laws of the United States, demonstrated by their continuous efforts to enter the country illegally.

The Assassination Attempts on Adolf Hitler.

Between 1921 and 1945, there were 32 documented accounts of the planned, attempted and failed assassination attempts made on the life of Adolf Hitler, the notorious Führer (Leader) of Nazi Germany. He was singularly responsible for the start of World War II and for the unspeakable crimes against humanity which resulted in the deaths of millions of people. Historically, very few people have been the intended target of as many assassination attempts as was Adolf Hitler.

Most of the early attempts on his life were spontaneous or poorly planned efforts by civilians who had little or no support from anyone or any organization. However, beginning in 1938, after Hitler had started grabbing territory in Europe, and for almost seven more years throughout World War II, members of the German elite began to plot against him. But for as long as Hitler and the Wehrmacht were winning battles, defeating nations, and occupying conquered territory, there was not much which the plotters could do. Hitler was too popular among the Germans to threaten.

Once Hitler made the flawed decision to break his Non-Aggression Pact with the Soviet Union and invade in June 1941, the fortunes of his Wehrmacht were reversed. Hitler continued to lose the confidence of more and more of his generals, many of whom he fired and replaced. The retreat from Moscow began Hitler's downfall, the demise of the Wehrmacht, and helped the plotters organize their most serious effort to assassinate him. The plan was to assassinate Hitler, seize power in Berlin, establish a new pro-Western government and save Germany from total defeat.

On July 20, 1944 Colonel Claus von Stauffenberg attended a meeting with Hitler and his senior officers in the Wolfsschanze (Wolf's Lair), one of Hitler's secure bunkers near the Eastern Front. There, he placed a briefcase containing plastic explosives under the table very close to where Hitler would be seated. Von Stauffenberg was outside the bunker when the explosives detonated. Wrongly, he assumed that Hitler and others had been killed and telephoned a report to that effect to other senior officers who were among the plotters in Germany and in occupied Europe.

But Hitler was not killed, only very seriously injured. Almost 5,000 persons were implicated in the assassination plot and executed. Hitler's favorite general, Field Marshal Erwin Rommel, the Desert Fox and Commander-in-Chief of the forces in Europe guarding against the Allied invasion, was forced to take poison. He once had told his friend, General Fritz Blumentritt, former Commander of a Corps and Army on the Western Front, that "The time has come when we must tell the Führer that we cannot continue the war."

Many of Hitler's senior officers and government officials, including two other field marshals, 19 generals, 26 colonels, two ambassadors, seven diplomats, and the Commander of the Berlin police committed suicide or were executed. Colonel Von Stauffenberg was executed by a firing squad on the night of the failed plot. Members of his family, friends, and close associates who were "guilty by association" were strung up with piano wire and hanged. Hitler had their deaths filmed. Tragically, in the nine months after the assassination plot failed, almost five million German citizens and soldiers perished. Add to that the incalculable number of Jews and other "untermenschen" (sub-humans) slaughtered in the frenzy of Hitler's "Final Solution" before the war ended in May 1945.

The courage of all the plotters against Hitler, intent upon eliminating the one person whose actions were bringing a once-great nation to ruin, was extraordinary. Today, in Berlin and elsewhere in Germany, monuments have been erected, and streets, parks and schools have been named in honor of the July 20th plotters.

This now is third example by people of character who put their lives on the line and risked death in order to defeat officious and oppressive rule by despotic governments. It should provide the impetus for ending all support for illegal immigration, for advocating that the people who compose the caravans, under the guise of fleeing oppression, return to their homelands. There they should demonstrate or fight for change. In the United States, taxpayer dollars should be spent on citizens who are in need, especially senior citizens and the handicapped whose needs tend to increase as they age.

"The best stories always end up being about the people rather than an event."

Stephen King, Author.

16. EPILOGUE

At the "DEDICATION" to this text is the statement, "I wrote this book hoping that the contents might give courage and strength to those who are battling this disease and to their families, friends and care providers who are with them and who are supporting them." Now, at end of almost 80,000 words, I believe that I have done that.

I thought it important to describe who we are as human beings, how we evolved, what makes us so very unique and so very special among all living things on the planet. I thought it important to understand in layman's terms what constitutes illness and disease, what is preventable and for what we may be predestined genetically. Similar to almost everything that we do in life, such as being a student, playing a sport, working a job, or raising a child, we do it all somewhat easier and often better when we have someone to help us. That is why I added the chapters about the roles of the family, medical community and care providers. The long "Chapter 14, DOROTHY, MY MOTHER," I hope satisfies the purpose of the dedication.

I know that many readers may wonder why I added "Chapter 15, RISE UP!", and what it has to do with helpful information for a person living with Parkinson's disease and the care providers. I added it to the narrative to raise the awareness of the reader that the United States of America has the intellectual and financial resources to improve dramatically the health care of its citizens most desperately in need of quality care. I want to live to see that happen and I will work for it.

Appendix 1. As I Start the Day.

This morning I begin another day. I am happy having the awareness that I will do things which are important in my life, and that I will do those things on my own to the best of my ability or with the support of people who love me and who I love. Everything that I accomplish today will give me the motivation and strength to continue to overcome challenges and enjoy life. I will do my best to keep to my daily routine knowing that it will make me strong in mind and in body.

Now I am ready to start my day.

Appendix 2. As I End the Day.

This evening I end another day. I am proud and happy about what I accomplished today by myself and with the help of people who support me and who love me. If I doubted myself for any reason, my faith in myself restored me. If I struggled, I did my best to recover. Everything that I did today was good for me and I am satisfied and happy. I look forward to another day tomorrow when I can continue to live as I am able and enjoy my life as I live it.

Appendix 3. I am the Caregiver.

Today I work for the benefit of a person in need. Together we are a team. Each of us is stronger as a part of that team. No task will be too great for either of us alone, but easier as we work together. Throughout our day, at all times I will be attentive, caring, compassionate, considerate, gentle, kind, and, most importantly loving. If, at the end of our day together, we have been productive and happy, then I know that I am a better person because of how we worked together and what we accomplished.

Appendix 4. Ad: Home Health Care Aide.

Home Health Care Aide needed at a private residence in Clear Lake for an elderly female, widowed, age 76, disabled by Parkinson's disease and osteoporosis. Height ~ 5'7" to 5'8" ; weight ~ 125 to 130 pounds. Individual is wheelchair-bound. Care is entirely within the home and on the property.

Hours are Monday through Friday, excluding Federal holidays, 7:30 a.m. to 12 noon and 1 p.m. to 6 p.m. daily.

Salary is $600. per week paid weekly. Paid vacation time at the same salary is for all U.S. Federal holidays, four days over the Easter holiday, two weeks during the summer, four days between Thanksgiving Day and the Sunday following Thanksgiving, and two weeks during the Christmas season from some time one week one before Christmas Day until one day after New Year's Day.

After two months' duty, one week's salary of $600. may be advanced for personal reasons. After four months' duty, two weeks' salary of $1,200. may be advanced for personal reasons.

There are two gentle, friendly dogs within the home: a medium-sized black Lab and a small Lhasa Apso.

Duties are entirely within the home or on the property.

Duties include:

- Morning transport from the bed to the wheelchair; transportation from the bedroom to the bathroom; transport from the wheelchair to and from the toilet; personal hygiene.
- Transportation from the bathroom to the kitchen for breakfast. (Table is pre-set and breakfast foods are prepared and located at the table or in the refrigerator).
- Companion time within the home or outdoors, weather permitting.
- During open / free time between 12:00 noon and 1 p.m. sponsor (son) is at home to bathe and dress his mother and walk the two dogs.
- Hot lunch at 1 p.m. (Table is pre-set and the lunch meal is prepared. When possible and convenient, lunch may be taken at a local restaurant. A credit card will be provided for the expenses.)
- Transportation from within the home to the kitchen for lunch.
- After lunch hygiene.
- Companion time within the home or outdoors, weather permitting.

A landline telephone and cellular telephone are available within the home for contact with the family members.

One bedroom furnished with a full-size bed, linens, two end tables and lamps, a dresser, a desk with desk light and closet; one full bathroom with toilet, tub, shower and double sink vanity; and, adjacent to the bedroom, a sitting room with closet, three-seat sofa, two-seat love seat, chair, end table, lamp, and flat screen television are available for the aide's private use.

If interested, please respond to this ad or flyer by e-mail to James Pelosi at: jjpelosi1973@att.net.

Please be willing to support an interview within the home and provide at least one current reference.

Appendix 5. EULOGY, MRS. DOROTHY PELOSI. Funeral Mass, St. Clare's Roman Catholic Church, Clear Lake, Texas, February 20, 2010. James Joseph Pelosi, son.

Good morning on this fine day.

Thank you all for taking the time this morning to come here to Saint Clare's to celebrate together the long and, to me, inspirational life of my mother Dorothy.

I would like start by offering a sincere "Thank You" to the priests, the staff and the parishioners here at St. Clare's for their support of my mother and me throughout the ten years that we tried to be faithful to the Mass schedule and, more importantly, for everything that they have done this week to support us once I became aware that this past Tuesday was at hand.

"Thank You" to our friends who always greeted Mom warmly whenever we met and who always asked about her status if she were not with me. A very special "Thank You" to Mrs. Arlene Cooley and Mrs. Carmel Garan, long-term friends here who helped today with the readings and whose support this week at our home I count among our many blessings.

Finally, I owe an exceptional "Thank You"

to Mrs. Deborah Schooley, mother of three grown sons, grandmother of an infant grandson, who was the primary caregiver for mother for most of the ten years that we were together. Long hours, irregular hours, difficult work which required a gentle, caring, and loving sentiment – Miss Deborah delivered on everything.

Mother and I were blessed to have Deborah within our home.

Now I briefly would like to reflect on the life of my mother which, to me, exemplified the best of all that is of value in life having lived 85 years dedicated and true to this faith; just over 60 years as a wife; just under 60 years as a mother; and right at 30 years as a grandmother.

Dorothy Muriel Hyacinth Rinderknecht was born on May 20th 1924 in one of the clustered suburbs of New York City. She was the second of two daughters, four years difference in age, part of what Tom Brokaw and most Americans acknowledge as "America's Greatest Generation."

Her mother for whom she had no childhood memories died when she was five. Her father held a variety of jobs. Money was tight especially during the depression of the 1930's as she was growing up.

More than once when the rent was unpaid, she walked from school to what she thought was home only to find what little there was of the family's property stacked on the street.

That family furniture included only one bed for four persons.

Mother told us that until she married our father at age 25 she never slept in her own bed. She and her sister traded places on a three-seat sofa or a two-seat piece of patio furniture which was kept indoors. They had blankets but no bedsheets.

She finished high school in June 1943.

She met my father at the end of WWII in 1945 after he returned from duty as a bomber pilot with the 8th Air Force.

She married him in January 1950.

Dad died two days before their 46th wedding anniversary. She wrote in her journal "I was proud to be his wife."

About ten years ago in 2000, Mother broke her hip which was re-set twice and never was able to respond to physical therapy. Less than six months later, she was diagnosed with Parkinson's disease which, combined with another diagnosis for osteoporosis, severely compromised her physically.

She lost the ability to use her legs and to walk, then to move her arms and to use her hands, to sense her comfort or discomfort and finally to communicate.

Fully aware of her disabilities none of us ever knew her to display any frustration or to express any anger at the crosses she carried. She believed that what happened in her life was God's will.

Two weeks before she died, she reduced her food intake by about half. A week before she died, she stopped eating completely including her regular dish of Blue Bell vanilla ice cream at lunch with Deborah and strawberry ice cream at supper with me.

Four days before she died, she stopped her intake of all fluids.

The day before she died Father Bob from this parish came to our home to administer the Sacrament of Healing.

Those of you who knew my mother and who had seen her within the past five years know that her elbows were locked into her sides; her forearms and hands were stiff against her chest; her fingers were locked into tight fists.

Father Bob recited his prayers. There was no indication that Mom had any awareness of the event. As Father Bob anointed her forehead, drawing with his thumb the sign of the cross and saying, "I absolve you in the name of the Father," my mother turned her head toward him, opened her fingers, and raised her hands and arms as if to embrace him.

Slowly my mother's body relaxed. All the rigidity from the Parkinson's receded like a wave from the shore. The pale, clammy appearance of her face was transformed to a soft rosy blush. The specs of calcium deposits which sprinkled isolated parts of her body evaporated. My two sisters and I were in awe.

My sense was that God's hand was on her and that His being was completely within her. Still, I keep asking myself "What is God's message here?"

Is there a message in how she lived her life?

Is there a message in her gracious acceptance of her disability and her handicaps?

Is there a message in her physical transformation one day before, at and beyond the hour of her death?

I cannot say that I think so. I am compelled to say that I know so. But it is not within my skill set to try to convey that message.

That is for Father Dominic and others like him and for each of us individually as we continue to live life, as we ask questions and as we seek answers.

Thank you all so very much. God Bless you, your families and all those who are closest to you.

God Bless you Mother. Thank you for giving me life and for sharing your wonderful life with us.

Be thou at peace.

APPENDIX 6. Parkinson's Disease Support Organizations in the United States.

The information provided at this Appendix is current as of the date of publication of this book, February 16, 2019.

The American Parkinson Disease Association (APDA) is a national network which provides information and referral, education and support programs, health and wellness activities, and events to help provide for a better quality of life for all persons within the Parkinson's community. Its motto is "Strength in optimism. Hope in progress."

The telephone number for its National Headquarters is 1-800-223-2732.

The support groups are free of charge and are for all persons living with Parkinson's disease, their spouses, family, friends and caregivers.

NATIONAL SUPPORT

Parkinson's Disease Advocate
Telephone: 551-482-7867

Parkinson's Disease Support Solutions
Telephone: 866-880-8582
www.parkinsonssupportsolutions.com

American Parkinson Disease Association (APDA)
Telephone: 800-223-2732
www.apdaparkinson.org

The Michael J. Fox Foundation for Parkinson's
Research
Telephone: 800-708-7644
www.michaeljfox.org

Parkinson's Disease Foundation (PDF)
Telephone. 800-457-6676
www.pdf.org

National Parkinson Disease Foundation
Telephone. 800-473-4636
www.parkinson.org

Parkinson's Disease Action Network
Telephone: 800-850-4726
www.parkinsonaction.org

The Caregiver Action Network
Telephone: 202-772-5050
www.caregiveraction.org

The Family Caregiver Alliance
Telephone: 800-445-8106
www.caregiver.org

STATE SUPPORT

ALABAMA
The University of Alabama
1720 7th Avenue South
Birmingham, AL 35294

ALASKA
The American Parkinson Disease Association
180 Nickerson Street
Suite 108
Seattle, WA 98109
Telephone: 206-695-2905

ARIZONA
The American Parkinson Disease Association
Post Office Box 40067
Tucson, AZ 85717-0067
Telephone: 206-695-2905

ARKANSAS
College of Medicine, University of Arkansas
Little Rock, Arkansas 72205
Telephone: 501-686-5270

CALIFORNIA
Information Center at Stanford University
300 Pasteur Drive, Room H-3144
Stanford, California 94305
Telephone: 650-724-6090

COLORADO
Colorado Parkinson Foundation, Inc
1155 Kelly Johnson Boulevard, Suite 111
Colorado Springs, Colorado 80920
Telephone: (719) 884-0103

CONNECTICUT
Information & Referral Center
Chase Family Movement Disorder Center
Ayer Neuroscience Institute
Hartford Healthcare
35 Talcottville Road, Suite 6
Vernon, CT 06066
Telephone: 860-490-5384

DELAWARE
450 South College Avenue or
The Star Building, 540 South College Avenue
Newark, Delaware, USA
Telephone: 302-354-5453

FLORIDA, North
Information & Referral Center
The Mayo Clinic, Jacksonville
4500 San Pablo Road
Jacksonville, FL 32224
Telephone:904-953-6096

FLORIDA, South
American Parkinson's Disease Association
700 West Hillsboro Blvd
Suite 3-110
Deerfield Beach, FL 33441
Telephone: 800-825-2732

GEORGIA
American Parkinson Disease Association, GA
Post Office Box 49416
Atlanta, GA 30359
Telephone: 404-325-2020

HAWAII
Hawaii Parkinson Association
P.O. Box 1312
Kailua, Hawaii 96734
Telephone: 808-219-8874

IDAHO
Idaho Department of Health & Welfare
Parkinson's Disease Information Center
1055 North Curtis Road
Boise, Idaho, 83706
Telephone: 208-367-6570

ILLINOIS
University of Chicago
Parkinson and Movement Disorder Clinic
5841 South Maryland Avenue
Chicago, Illinois 60637
Telephone: 773-702-1220

INDIANA
Indiana Parkinson Foundation
14350 Mundy Drive Suite 800 #181,
Noblesville, IN 46060
Telephone: 317-550-5648

IOWA
Parkinson's Information and Referral Center
1200 Pleasant Street, E524
Des Moines, Iowa 50309
Telephone: 515-241-6379

KANSAS
The University of Kansas Medical Center
3901 Rainbow Boulevard
Kansas City, KS 66160
Telephone 913-588-5000

LOUISIANA
Louisiana Services Network Data Consortium
Parkinson's Disease Support
LSU Health Science Center
Department of Neurology
1501 Kings Highway
Shreveport, LA 71103
Telephone: (318) 675-6142

MAINE
Stephens Memorial Hospital
181 Main Street
Norway, Maine 04268
Telephone: 207-743-5933

MARYLAND
University of Maryland
110 S Paca Street, 3rd Floor
Baltimore, MD 21201
Telephone: 410-328-333

MASSACHUSETTS
Information & Referral Center
Boston University School of Medicine
72 East Concord Street, Room C3
Boston, MA 02118
Telephones: 617-638-8466 and 800-651-8466

MICHIGAN
Michigan Parkinson Foundation
30400 Telegraph Road, Suite 150
Bingham Farms, MI 48025
Telephones: 248-433-1011 and 800-852-9781

MINNESOTA
Abbott Northwestern Hospital
MR 12209
800 E 28th St.
Minneapolis, MN 55407
Telephone: 651-241-8297

MISSISSIPPI
1040 River Oaks Drive
Flowood, MS 39232
Toll-free telephone: 800-223-2732

MISSOURI
The American Parkinson Disease Association
Resources & Support
1415 Elbridge Payne Road, Suite 150
Chesterfield, Missouri 63017
Telephone: 636-778-3377

MONTANA
Department of Public Health and Human Services
500 W Broadway St
Missoula, MT 59802
Telephone: 406-251-5338

NEBRASKA
Parkinson's Nebraska
16811 Burdette St., Suite 1
Omaha, NE 68116
Telephone: 402-715-4707
info@parkinsonsnebraska.org

NEVADA
Parkinson's Disease Information Center
975 Kirman Avenue
Reno, NV 89502-0993
Telephone: 775-328-1715

NEW HAMPSHIRE
Parkinson's Disease and Movement
Disorders Resource Center
Lebanon, NH (DHMC)
Telephone: 603-653-6672

NEW JERSEY
APDA Information & Referral Center
Robert Wood Johnson Wellness Center
Wellness Plaza
100 Kirkpatrick Street, 2nd Floor
New Brunswick, NJ 08901
Telephone: 732-745-7320, extension #1

NEW YORK
Parkinson's Disease Foundation, Inc.
1359 Broadway, Suite 1509
New York, New York 10018
Telephone: New York: 212-457-6676
Toll-free telephone:800-457-6676
URL: http://www.pdf.org

NORTH CAROLINA
Parkinson Association of the Carolinas
2101 Sardis Road North, Box 15
Charlotte, NC 28227
Telephone: 704-248-3722
Toll-free telephone: 866-903-PARK (7275)
Email: pac@parkinsonassociation.org

NORTH DAKOTA
Marv Bossart Foundation for Parkinson's
Support.
4141 28th Ave South
Fargo, ND 58104
Telephone: 701-371-3196
email: info@marvbossartfoundation.org

OHIO
The Parkinson Foundation
2800 Corporate Exchange Drive, Suite 360
Columbus, OH 43231
Telephone: 614-890-1901
Toll-free telephone: 866-920-6673
Email: ohioinfo@parkinson.org

OKLAHOMA
Parkinson Foundation of Oklahoma
OKC OFFICE
720 W. Wilshire, Suite 109
Oklahoma City, OK 73116
Telephone: 405-810-0695

OREGON
Parkinson's Resources of Oregon
8880 SW Nimbus Avenue, Suite B
Beaverton, OR 97008
Helpline: 503-594-0901 or 800-426-6806
email: info@parkinsonsresources.org

PENNSYLVANIA
Mail Code H109, Room C2846
500 University Drive, PO Box 850
Hershey, PA 17033-0850
Telephone: 717-531-3598

RHODE ISLAND
Post Office Box 41659
Providence, RI 02940
Telephone: 401-736-1046
Email: apdari@apdaparkinson.org

SOUTH CAROLINA
Columbia Parkinson's Support Group
P.O. Box 1393
Columbia, SC 29202
Telephone: 803-335-4247 (10 a.m.- 8 p.m.)
www.columbiaparkinsonsupportgroup.org

SOUTH DAKOTA
South Dakota Parkinson Foundation
1000 N West Ave, Suite 220
Sioux Falls, SD 57104
Telephone: 605-271-6113

TENNESSEE
Vanderbilt University Medical Center
1211 Medical Center Drive
Nashville, TN 37232
Telephone: 615-322-5000
Telephone: 615-936-0060

TEXAS
The American Parkinson Disease Association
Resources & Support
22211 IH10W, Suite 2101
San Antonio, TX 78257
Telephone: 210-580-3416

UTAH
Bureau of Health Promotion
Utah Department of Health
Salt Lake City, UT 84114-2107
Telephone: 801-538-6244
Email: mfriedrichs@utah.gov

VERMONT
UVM Medical Center
1 South Prospect St.
Burlington VT 05401
Telephone: 802-847-3366

VIRGINIA
The American Parkinson Disease Association
Center of Virginia
Post Office Box 801018
Charlottesville, VA 22908
Telephone: 434-982-4482
e-mail: sjd3c@virginia.edu

WASHINGTON
The American Parkinson Disease Association
180 Nickerson Street, Suite 108
Seattle, WA 98109
Telephone: 206-695-2905

WEST VIRGINIA
West Virginia Parkinson's Support
222 Capitol Street, Suite 400
Charleston, WV 25301
Telephone: 304-343-2800
e-mail: manahan@aol.com

WISCONSIN
The American Parkinson Disease Association
5900 Monona Drive, Suite 407
Monona, WI 53716
Telephone: 608-345-7938

Wisconsin Parkinson Association
16655 W. Bluemound Road, Suite 330
Brookfield, WI 53005
Telephone: 414.312.6990
e-mail: www.wiparkinson.org

WYOMING
Wyoming Medical Center
1233 E. Second St.
Casper, WY 82601
Telephone: 307-577-7201
Toll-free telephone: 800-822-7201

APPENDIX 7. Parkinson's Disease Support Organizations in Canada.

PARKINSON CANADA

https://www.parkinson.ca

Since 1965, *Parkinson Canada* has been the national advocate for Canadians who are living with Parkinson's disease and for their spouses, family, friends, coworkers and others who are supporting them. *Parkinson Canada* provides education and support services to everyone joined in the battle against Parkinson's disease.

Parkinson Canada is accredited by Imagine Canada's Standards program, recognizing a quality of excellence in five fundamental areas: board governance, financial accountability and transparency, fundraising, staff management, and volunteer involvement.

Parkinson Canada promotes issues that are relevant and important to the members of the Parkinson's community through interaction with the Canadian federal, provincial and territorial governments. The *Parkinson Canada* Research Program funds innovative research to search for advanced and improved treatments therapies and a cure.

At the "Message from our CEO," *Parkinson*

Canada Chief Executive Officer, Ms. Joyce Gordon, wrote at the website to the Parkinson community announcing that:

- *Parkinson Canada* is an online resource to Canada's Parkinson's community for information describing resources and support for anyone living with Parkinson's. One resource is the book, *"Parkinson's Disease: An Introductory Guide"* by Doctors Ron Postuma and Julius Anang in collaboration with McGill University Health Centre. The second resource is another book, "Medications to Treat Parkinson's Disease," developed by pharmacists for both health professionals and members of the Parkinson's community.

- Keeping informed about the disease is one of the best tools to living well. *Parkinson Canada* hosts webinars and podcasts on its Knowledge Network. Past webinar presentations also are available for replay on the *Parkinson Canada* YouTube channel. Past podcasts can be accessed from SoundCloud.

- *Parkinson Canada* supports a Medical Advisory Committee with experts in a variety of fields who are knowledgeable about the latest information concerning Parkinson's disease.

Parkinson Canada
Charitable Registration Number:
10809 – 1786 – RR0001
4211 Yonge Street, Suite 31
Toronto, ON M2P 2A9
Telephone: 416-227-9700
Toll-free: 1-800-565-3000

APPENDIX 8. Parkinson's Disease Support Organizations in Europe.

European Parkinson's Disease Association
1 Cobden Road
Sevenoaks, Kent TN13 3UB
United Kingdom
info@epda.eu.com

The European Parkinson's Disease Association announces at its website that it is the only European Parkinson's oversight and sponsorship organisation and working with the Parkinson's community for 25 years. It provides information and resources to all persons living with Parkinson's disease, their spouses, family, and friends. Its vision is to enable all people with Parkinson's to live a full life and to support the search for a cure.

The European Parkinson's Disease Association represents the national Parkinson's Disease Associations in nearly 30 countries with 120,000 members across Europe. It serves as an advocate for the rights and needs of more than 1.2 million people living with Parkinson's disease and their families.

BELGIUM
Vlaamse Parkinson Liga vzw
Diestsevest 33 bus 302
3000 Leuven
Belgium
e-mail: info@parkinsonliga.be
website: www.parkinsonliga.be
FB: www.facebook.com/groups/290945381111324

CROATIA
CR Udruga Parkinson i mi
Crnatkova 18
10 000 Zagreb Croatia
e-mail: parkinsonimi@gmail.com website
website: http://parkinsonimi.com/
facebook: www.facebook.com/ParkinsonIMi

THE CZECH REPUBLIC
Společnost PARKINSON, z. s
Czech Parkinson's Disease Society
Volyňská 20
Praha 10   100 00
Czech Republic
e-mail: kancelar@spolecnost-parkinson.cz
website: www.spolecnost-parkinson.cz
website: www.parkinson-brno.cz
FB: www.facebook.com/spolecnostparkinson

DENMARK
Parkinsonforeningen
The Danish Parkinson Association
Blekinge Boulevard 2
2630 Taastrup
Denmark
e-mail: info@parkinson.dk
website www.parkinson.dk
FB: www.facebook.com/Parkinsonforeningen

ESTONIA
Eesti Parkinsoniliit
Estonian Parkinson's Association
Endla 59
Tallin Harjumaa
10615 Estonia
Website: www.parkinson.ee
FB: www.facebook.com/Eesti-Parkinsoniliit-
167882163562086

FINLAND
Erityisosaamiskeskus Suvituuli
(Rehabilitation Centre)
Suvilinnantie 2
PL 905 FI-20101
Turku, Finland
e-mail: parkinson-liitto@parkinson.fi
website: www.parkinson.fi
facebook: www.facebook.com/parkinsonfi
twitter: @Parkinsonliitto

FRANCE
Association France Parkinson
18 rue des terres au curé
75013 Paris France
e-mail: infos@franceparkinson.fr
website: www.franceparkinson.fr
FB: www.facebook.com/chaquepasestuneconquete
twitter: @FranceParkinson

GREECE
ΕΠΙΚΟΥΡΟΣ - κίνηση
EPIKOUROS - Kinesis (Movement) Branch
Leoforos Galatsioy 127
Athens 11146 Greece
e-mail: info@parkinsonportal.gr
website: www.parkinsonportal.gr
FB:www.facebook.com/Parkinson.EPIKOYROS.kinesis

HUNGARY
Delta Magyar Parkinson Egyesület
Delta Hungarian Parkinson's Association
Balassa 6
Budapest H-1083 Hungary
e-mail: info@fogomakezed.hu
website: www.fogomakezed.hu

ICELAND
PSÍ - Parkinsonsamtökin á Íslandi
Hátúni 10b
IS-105 Reykjavík Iceland
e-mail: parkinsonsamtokin@gmail.com
website www.parkinson.is
facebook: www.facebook.com/parkinsonsamtokin

IRELAND
Parkinson's Association of Ireland
Carmichael House
North Brunswick Street
Dublin 7 Ireland
e-mail: info@parkinsons.ie website
www.parkinsons.ie
FB: www.facebook.com/parkinsons.ireland
twitter: @ParkinsonsIre

ITALY
Parkinson Italia (ONLUS)
Confederazione Associazioni Italiane
Parkinson E Parkinsonism
Via San Vittore 16
20123 Milano Italy
e-mail: segreteria@parkinson-italia.it
website: www.parkinson-italia.it
FB:www.facebook.com/parkinsonitaliaonlus.it
Twitter: @ParKinsonITALY

LITHUANIA
Lietuvos Parkinsono ligos draugija
Lithuanian Parkinson's Disease Society
Naujakiemio str. 17B
Vilnius LT-08314 Lithuania
Website: www.parkinsonas.org
FB: facebook www.facebook.com/Lietuvos-
Parkinsono-ligos-draugija-1644805589108057

LUXEMBOURG
Parkinson Luxembourg (PL) a.s.b.l
16, rue des Champs
BP 1348
Leudelange 3348 Luxembourg
e-mail: info@parkinsonlux.lu
website: www.parkinsonlux.lu
facebook: www.facebook.com/parkinsonlux

MALTA
Malta Parkinson's Disease Association
P.O. Box 17
Marsa MTP 1001 Malta
e-mail: info@maltaparkinsons.com
website: www.maltaparkinsons.com
FB:www.facebook.com/MaltaParkinsonsDiseaseAssociation

THE NETHERLANDS
Parkinson Vereniging (PV)
Kosterijland 12
Postbus 46
Bunnik 3981 AJ Netherlands
Email: info@parkinson-vereniging.nl
website www.parkinson-vereniging.nl
FB:www.facebook.com/parkinsonvereniging
twitter: @Parkinson_NL

NORWAY
Norges Parkinsonforbund
Norwegian Parkinson's Disease Association
Karl Johansgate 7
0154 Oslo Norway
e-mail: post@parkinson.no
website: www.parkinson.no
facebook:www.facebook.com/NorgesParkinsonforbund
twitter: @NorgesParkinson

POLAND
Krakowskie Stowarzyszenie Osób Dotkniętych
Chorobą Parkinsona
Kraków Parkinson's Disease Association
ul. Mikołajska 2
31-027 Kraków Poland
e-mail: ksodchp@parkinson.krakow.pl
website: www.parkinson.krakow.

PORTUGAL
Associação Portuguesa de Doentes de
Parkinson - APDPk
Bairro da Liberdade
lote 11, loja 17
1070 - 023 Lisboa Portugal
e-mail: secretariadoparkinson@gmail.com
website: www.parkinson.pt
facebook: www.facebook.com/APDPK
facebook: www.facebook.com/lisboa.parkinson

SLOVENIA
Društvo TREPETLIKA
Parkinson's Disease Society of Slovenia
Šišenska cesta 23
Ljubljana 1000 Slovenija
e-mail: trepetlikadrustvo@gmail.com
website: www.trepetlika.si
facebook www.facebook.com/drustvotrepetlika
twitter: @drustvotrep

SPAIN
Federación Española de Párkinson
Spanish Federation of Parkinson Disease
Paseo Ermita del Santo
5, 1ª planta, oficina 1F
Madrid 28011 Spain
e-mail: info@esparkinson.es
website: www.esparkinson.es
FB:www.facebook.com/federacionespanoladeparkinson
twitter: @ParkinsonFEP

SWEDEN
ParkinsonFörbundet
The Swedish Parkinson's Disease Association
Skeppargatan 52
Stockholm 11458 Sweden
e-mail: parkinsonforbundet@telia.com
website: www.parkinsonforbundet.se
FB: www.facebook.com/Parkinsonforbundet

SWITZERLAND
Parkinson Schweiz
Gewerbestrasse 12a
Postfach 123
Egg Zürich 8132 Switzerland
e-mail: info@parkinson.ch
website: www.parkinson.ch
facebook: www.facebook.com/ParkinsonSchweiz

UKRAINE
Ukrainian Parkinson Disease Society
Institute of Gerontology
Vyshgorodskaya Street 67
Natl Academy of Science
04114 Kiev Ukraine
e-mail: kin@geront.kiev.ua
website: www.geront.kiev.ua

ABOUT THE AUTHOR

James Joseph Pelosi is a former Army officer, university professor and aerospace engineer retired with 42 years government service. He earned a Bachelor of Science degree in Civil and Mechanical engineering from the United States Military Academy at West Point, New York with the "Proud and Free" class of 1973; a Master in Business Administration degree from Pepperdine University's Presidential and Key Executive program in Los Angeles, California in 1982; a Master of Arts degree in Russian Area Studies from Georgetown University's overseas extension program at the U.S. Army Russian Institute in Garmisch-Partenkirchen, Germany in 1985; and a Doctor of Philosophy degree in Aerospace Biomedical Engineering from Moscow State University, Russia in 1988. He spends his time conducting research for future publications and as a volunteer for medical research investigations related to healthy aging. He resides among residences in the United States, Germany, Italy and Russia. His first book, *Normandy to Berlin: The Trek to Honor the Legacies*, describes his 59-day, 895-mile walk between Omaha Beach, Normandy, France and the Brandenburg Gate, Berlin, Germany in 2014. Available at amazon.com.

All profits from the sale of that book are donated to combat-wounded disabled veterans.

He is a 39-year member of the American Legion and an advocate for all veterans especially those disabled by combat.

All profits from the sale of this book are donated to persons living with Parkinson's disease especially those veterans who also have suffered traumatic brain injuries.

JAMES JOSEPH PELOSI

CPSIA information can be obtained
at www.ICGtesting.com
Printed in the USA
LVHW011651250319
611743LV00002B/418/P